T0329894

Maya Bonesetters

Maya Bonesetters

Manual Healers in a Changing Guatemala

SERVANDO Z. HINOJOSA
ILLUSTRATIONS BY SERVANDO G. HINOJOSA

University of Texas Press ◆ *Austin*

Requests for permission to reproduce material from this work should be sent to:
  Permissions
  University of Texas Press
  P.O. Box 7819
  Austin, TX 78713-7819
  utpress.utexas.edu/rp-form

The line drawings are courtesy of the artist, Servando G. Hinojosa.

♾ The paper used in this book meets the minimum requirements of ANSI/NISO Z39.48-1992 (R1997) (Permanence of Paper).

An earlier version of chapter 4 appeared in "Bonesetting and Radiography in the Southern Maya Highlands," *Medical Anthropology* 23, no. 4 (2004). Reprinted by permission of the publisher, Taylor & Francis, https://www.tandfonline.com. Earlier versions of other material appeared in "'The Hands Know': Bodily Engagement and Medical Impasse in Highland Maya Bonesetting," *Medical Anthropology Quarterly* 16, no. 1 (March 2002).

Library of Congress Cataloging-in-Publication Data
Names: Hinojosa, Servando Z., 1968– author.
Title: Maya bonesetters : manual healers in a changing Guatemala / Servando Hinojosa.
Description: First edition. | Austin : University of Texas Press, 2020. | Includes bibliographical references and index.
Identifiers: LCCN 2019021577 | ISBN 978-1-4773-2029-7 (paperback) | ISBN 978-1-4773-2028-0 (cloth) | ISBN 978-1-4773-2030-3 (library ebook) | ISBN 978-1-4773-2031-0 (nonlibrary ebook)
Subjects: LCSH: Bonesetters—Guatemala. | Maya healers—Guatemala. | Manipulation (Therapeutics)—Guatemala. | Mayas—Medicine—Guatemala. | Traditional medicine—Guatemala.
Classification: LCC F1465.3.M4 H56 2020 | DDC 972.81—dc23
LC record available at https://lccn.loc.gov/2019021577

doi:10.7560/320280

Contents

Preface and Acknowledgments

What prompted this work about Maya bonesetters? First, there was personal interest, and then I realized that there were big gaps in the literature when it came to these specialists. This made me wonder why anthropologists had not written very much about bonesetters. We pay attention, after all, to how people define sickness and get healed when they are sick, so it puzzled me that such a large domain of the treatment of infirmity — injury and other physical limitations — had attracted so little attention. One possibility is that researchers simply preferred learning about better-known kinds of healers and ritualists. I, too, was first drawn to the work of midwives, ceremonial dancers, and spiritual healers before I shifted most of my focus to bonesetters. The bonesetters' work has not received much attention in the public health field, either, perhaps because what bonesetters do is somewhat hard to scale and measure. As a result, bonesetters have been largely excluded from conversations about traditional health practitioners and community health resources, and when they have appeared in some medical literature it has reflected anything but their best work. Given how bonesetters have been routinely excluded from the pages of ethnographies, one could be forgiven for concluding that bonesetters simply have no place in the researcher's notebooks. Or one might not even notice their absence at all. I wrote this book in part to remedy these silences.

I first wrote about Maya bonesetters while carrying out my master's research in 1992 and 1993 in San Juan Comalapa, then put it aside. When I was able to return to this research, progress was often very slow: I could not quite figure out how to approach the bonesetters' work, and there were few published works to guide me. But it was clear that bonesetters mattered to local people. In Comalapa, San Pedro La Laguna, and San Juan La

Laguna, bonesetters mobilize around the unexpected. They are often called to the front lines when injury happens, and they continue helping the injured with follow-up care. A Maya bonesetter tries to return bodies to a normative state using a palette of techniques not only unique to him or her as an individual but often unique to specific communities as well. And even if bonesetters are not visible in communities, there is nearly always a bonesetter at work there somewhere, much as bonesetters of other traditions are at work in virtually every corner of the world. No matter the culture, different kinds of bonesetters labor behind the scenes to ease the physical pains and limitations that people deal with, even more so in areas with few formal health resources. Their work seldom gets acknowledged, though, whether in highland Guatemala or in other parts of the world.

It does not help that Guatemalan Maya bonesetters generally do not identify with each other as practitioners or see each other as part of a group, because this probably reduces their visibility even more. That they express little to no group identity surprised me at first, as did the finding that bonesetters do not treat each other with collegiality and do not refer clients to each other.[1] I was also surprised to learn that the bonesetters were almost all self-taught; they seldom mentioned learning from another bonesetter's examples, much less learning from another bonesetter's direct teachings. In the years since I began paying attention to Maya bonesetters, in fact, their status as independent workers has been a recurring theme. Even if the bonesetters might foster a kind of social cohesion when they are treating people, with their work bringing neighbors together in times of crisis, ironically the bonesetters do not engender similar ties among each other.

However few ties might bind them to each other, Maya bonesetters are undeniably there for other people. In Guatemala—whether they call themselves *hueseros, componehuesos, jaladores de huesos, arregladores de huesos, curanderos,* or *wikol baq*—they labor to get people back on their feet and back to their normal life roles. Bonesetters do this, moreover, fully aware that if a client is not satisfied with the care he or she receives from a particular bonesetter, the client might move on to another bonesetter, or maybe even to a clinician. Bonesetters thus work in a context in which clients can choose to discontinue seeing them, reminding us that not only do sufferers exercise some choice of caregiver, but they remain the final arbiters about how their bodies get handled. They actively seek care while preserving sovereignty over their bodies.

As Maya care-seekers know, Maya bonesetters work in different ways, and these differences have in turn affected the scaffolding of this book. The chapters that follow reflect how bonesetters of the first town where I conducted research, San Juan Comalapa, utilize a fully empirical approach, whereas bonesetters of the other two towns, San Pedro La Laguna and San Juan La Laguna, pair their manual techniques with sacred elements. Bonesetters of these two broad areas cleave tightly to their own ways of treating bodies, in a manner emblematic of how many variations can develop within specific fields of traditional medicine, even among those fields practiced by closely related cultural groups. As different as these expressions of bonesetting may be from one another, they both exist in a landscape of changing risks and resources. In recent decades, they have had to face many challenges to their way of operating.

To understand these bonesetting traditions' relevance to Maya lives today, I have needed to situate them within the current lived landscape of Guatemala, including the lived medical landscape. For this reason I made the study multisited, both spatially and structurally, moving between the popular and formal health sectors and engaging with clinicians whenever possible. In the process it became immediately apparent that even though clinicians hold more economic and political sway than do Maya bonesetters, biomedicine as a whole has not eclipsed bonesetting. Bonesetters still command a lot of respect from people in general, something that probably has to do both with how they maintain a certain autonomy from the health system and with how they actually treat people. And just as most physicians express a great deal of apprehension about Maya bonesetters, individuals they consider unfit to treat others, bonesetters also voice many reservations about physicians. This state of affairs makes it unlikely that some kind of productive interaction between these different practitioners can occur in the near future, at least in Guatemala, but it does not mean the end of the road for Maya bonesetters. Guatemalans keep getting injured, and many of those that do will keep finding their way to those humble homes in their neighborhoods where bonesetters will put aside whatever they are doing and try to help them.

When I began this work over twenty-five years ago, I had no idea what final form it would eventually take. But as it stands now, this study, with all its lacunae, represents merely one step toward putting bonesetters firmly into conversations about traditional medicine specialists and the changes they are facing. I am not sure whether bonesetting will ever get moved into broader usage in Guatemala, but it is clear that wider acceptance will have to rest upon a broader appreciation of indigenous knowledge in general. Bonesetting's acceptance will ultimately need to hinge on a growing recognition that indigenous people have much to contribute to discussions of health, even when so much of the health system's own attention is focused on advanced technologies. In the meantime, Maya bonesetters continue to work, to adapt, and to keep as much of their character as possible. They have been anything but static over the years, responding to changes and opportunities while valuing a tradition whose last act is yet to be written. And though this book still leaves many areas yet to explore, I hope it will shed a little light on the universal store of knowledge that bonesetters have been building for so long.

Acknowledgments

As so often happens with ethnographic works, especially with those that take as long as this one, far more people have lent a supportive hand than I can properly thank. My mind immediately goes to my friend and mentor Judith Maxwell, who in 1990 helped launch what became my research career in Guatemala. I am also indebted to Victoria Bricker and the late Munro Edmonson, both of Tulane University, for walking me through the many chapters and permutations of Middle America. I recall with gratitude the late Ben Paul and his early work with Lake Atitlán bonesetters. His encouragement, when I was just finding my research footing, gave me a renewed sense of purpose.

In Guatemala many thanks go to Chuti' Hunahpu' and his late mother, Herlinda, for introducing me to Kaqchikel Maya bonesetters when they were first opening their San Juan Comalapa home to me. Other friends and families in Comalapa always made me feel welcome and eager to return. In San Pedro La Laguna, meanwhile, Ajpub' Pablo García Ixmata' and his father opened many doors for me, for which I am very grateful. Ajpub' made it possible for me to meet Tz'utujiil Maya bonesetters he knew directly and indirectly, and these became the core group of bonesetters I worked with in the Lake Atitlán area.

Despite the misgivings many physicians have about bonesetters, my conversations with them reminded me how injury can benefit from the talents of different kinds of health practitioners. I value their frankness. I also appreciate those Guatemalan physicians whom I spoke with over the years but who, because we did not specifically talk about bonesetters, are not included in this book.

Those who deserve the most credit for this work, of course, are the bonesetters of San Juan Comalapa, San Pedro La Laguna, and San Juan La Laguna and the people they introduced me to. Without their interest and willingness to let me enter their healing spaces, hear their stories, learn from them, and ask questions, none of this work could have been possible. I have tried to capture their individual voices with quotes whenever possible, using their rural variants of Guatemalan Spanish. People such as these bonesetters remind me why people need local healers as much as they need clinicians—each brings something unique to the larger whole that is a care-seeker. The bonesetters of these three towns have kept me in admiration of the bonesetting craft and its unfinished history, and I just hope I have represented them with the appreciation and grace they deserve.

Most bonesetters and other individuals in this work are referred to using pseudonyms, both because of a respect for privacy and largely because the political climate in Guatemala, even following the 1996 Peace Accords, advises caution with using the identities of local people. The only persons whose names I have included in the text are those of Hugo Icú Perén, a health practitioner and senior administrator at a community health association, and the late Alejandro Chacach, who was a dear friend and whose family appreciates the lasting effects of his healing work.

A later phase of this research received support from the Foundation for the Advancement of Mesoamerican Studies, Inc. (FAMSI), which I gratefully acknowledge. This comprised grants in 2000 (No. 99018) and 2001 (No. 00036). All errors in fact or interpretation are fully my own and in no way reflect the position of FAMSI. I likewise thank the journal *Medical Anthropology Quarterly* for the material I have adapted here from an article published in 2002. For allowing me to reuse much of an article published in 2004, which I have expanded considerably for this book, I also express my deepest appreciation to the editors of the journal *Medical Anthropology*. I offer my thanks as well to Mirela Conner for permitting me to use a photograph she took of a public mural in San Juan La Laguna.

Great appreciation goes to Sheila Cosminsky, who read an earlier version of this manuscript and offered very constructive feedback. Hers is a voice that I hold in highest esteem. To my friend and colleague Kathryn S. Oths, I also extend my appreciation for early on validating my interest in bonesetters. Fortunately for me, it was an interest that she shared and that we were able to develop into an edited volume about bonesetters published in 2004. My sincere thanks also go to the anonymous reader who gave me excellent suggestions on improving the manuscript for this book. He or she attuned me to the need to elaborate further on how physicians and bonesetters regard each other, and to pay closer attention to what health centers can reveal about the way people do or do not report injuries to them. This recommendation allowed me to buttress some of my findings with multiyear quantitative public data from two communities.

Casey Kittrell of the University of Texas Press deserves great credit for shepherding the manuscript through the entire editorial process. His steadfast belief in the value of this work, together with his editorial expertise, made a huge difference in bringing the overall project to completion. My thanks go also to copyeditor Sonya Manes for her very discerning eyes. It has been a great privilege working with her and with all the members of the University of Texas Press editorial team.

For making the visual dimension of the work possible, there is no one I can thank more than my father, Servando G. Hinojosa. Even when the tasks of crafting the bonesetter portraits and of skillfully re-creating the treatment scenes were too much for me to envision, he worked on them, one pen stroke at a time. He put many of my ideas about movement and composition into artistic form and into the lived settings I described to him, something he has done beautifully every time I have asked him to illustrate a book for me. The portraits he made of several now-deceased bonesetters still stir me, and speak more poignantly about them than my accounts of their life and work do. For her continuous moral support during the many years that this project has taken, I also thank my mother, Petra Z. Hinojosa. And for their boundless humor and hospitality over the years, I send my best to my in-laws Turker and Yuksel Kayaardı, as well as to Mark and Diana Glazer.

At the end of the day, there has been no greater source of support and encouragement than my wife, Nihan Kayaardı-Hinojosa. Together with our daughter, Asya Mia, she remains a most steadying presence in my life, and someone with whom I am only too grateful to share the lively transatlantic world we inhabit.

Maya Bonesetters

Introduction

I was a bit surprised when Lázaro asked me to duck. We were standing in a room where Lázaro was treating someone with an injured wrist and hip, when one of the men with us, who had been looking outside the window, quickly closed the curtain and whispered something. Someone switched off the lights, and the room went quiet. Even the middle-aged man who seconds before had been receiving treatment lay quietly on the bed. A moment later someone appeared at the window, their figure outlined in the early morning sun reaching through the thin drapes. We looked at each other as the knocking began. I knew better than to ask who was at the door, but still wondered about who could cause such a commotion. Was it a local physician who had heard that Lázaro, a Maya bonesetter, was making a house call? Or was it someone the injured man owed money to? After a couple of minutes, when the person at the door stopped knocking and moved on, one man cautiously edged the curtain aside and looked down the street. He gave the all clear. We got up from the floor, and Lázaro once again leaned over the man on the bed and continued treating him. It was not until later that morning that Lázaro, no doubt sensing how puzzled I was, told me what had happened, and who had been at the door. Had he explained that it had been a bill collector, or even an estranged relative, I might have understood why we needed to react as we did. The last thing I expected for him to say was that it had been another Maya bonesetter.

This was one of the times during my research on Maya bonesetters that I saw, during what I thought was a typical treatment encounter, something unexpected, a point of tension. On this day I was reminded that while Maya bonesetters do as much as they can to treat their clients, they do not usually abide one another. In fact, I have never known one Maya bonesetter to refer a client to another bonesetter, or even to acknowledge much skill in another bonesetter. This marked one instance in which a bone-setter averted an embarrassing face-to-face with another bonesetter, par-ticularly since the client had earlier been treated four times by the bone-setter who came knocking at the door and who was expected to arrive at the house on that day. For his part, Lázaro accepted the injured man as a client, knowing that he would have to work with a body that already bore the effects of previous treatment. Lázaro had been in this situation many times before, but usually with clients who had gone to clinicians, not to bonesetters, before they came to him.

Lázaro had learned how to handle situations such as this in the same way that he learned to set bones: he simply taught himself. As most bone-setters say about themselves, Lázaro said he was self-taught, and whether or not this played into his poor regard for other bonesetters, his mode of learning challenged an assumption I tacitly carried when I began my field-work. I had expected that individuals who were to become bonesetters would first spend years observing and assisting experienced bonesetters before they would get recognized as bonesetters in their own right. What I nearly always found, though, was that instead of being trained through prolonged apprenticeships, bonesetters entered the craft out of sheer ne-cessity. They found themselves suddenly having to help others, whether or not they had any proven skill. Those who did show some skill and got good results would likely be talked about by others. And the more people talked about them, the more others would hear about them. Their reputa-tion would soon bring people to their door.

I did not know much about Maya bonesetters when I started because, in spite of how integral their work is to Maya communities, few people have written about them. Theirs may be a widespread and essential activity, but it is still very underdocumented, something that surprised me, as it no doubt might surprise others familiar with ethnographic works written about Mayas or about other Mesoamerican groups. Those familiar with studies of twentieth-century Mayas would recognize that while much re-search has centered on the healing traditions of midwifery, ethnobotany, shamanism, and even daykeeping, little has centered on bonesetting. It is almost as if bonesetting fell outside the scope of both community-based ethnography and medical anthropology, or as if it did not measure up to the importance enjoyed by other Maya diagnostic and healing traditions. It is tempting to say that researchers have not been drawn to Maya bone-setting because, in its most general expressions, it is not deeply mysti-cal or heavy with spiritual meaning. Bonesetting, rather, has more to do with physical diagnoses, manipulations, and restoration of bodily well-being and movement. Whatever the case, bonesetting has attracted the attention of few anthropologists, which represents a great omission in our efforts to learn about Mayas.

By focusing on Maya bonesetting, then, this book represents a step away from conversations about cloistered mystical practices and a step toward talking about daily life. I intend not so much to analyze the efficacy of bonesetting treatments as to frame some of the cultural meanings of the craft. Because Maya bonesetting remains so little explored and so often disparaged by biomedicine, part of my task is to point out that bonesetting comprises a valued set of activities that developed long before understandings of Western medicine and surgery took their present forms. As I explore in later chapters, bonesetting traditions emerged everywhere in the world because people everywhere get injured. But bonesetting's very antiquity has made it subject to criticism by Western medical voices, which largely dismiss its legitimacy and reject its methods.

Chief among the criticisms biomedicine levels against Maya bonesetting is the idea that non–medically trained individuals can diagnose and treat using nothing but their hands. Applying their hands to suffering bodies, bonesetters manifest a body-based knowledge relying on an untaught, nonbiomedical empathy, an approach that does not sit well with Western medical practitioners. Still, since few Mayas and even fewer Maya bonesetters are in a position to challenge biomedical authority, they have few options but to keep a low profile if they want to avoid problems. Biomedicine casts a long shadow everywhere in Guatemala, though, creating an uneasy situation for bonesetters, who are approached almost every day by people needing help. In the end, bonesetters try to help people not because local institutions do or do not favor them, but simply because they feel bound to help. They also worry about what might happen to those people if they go to someone else for care.

As I saw when I was with Lázaro, Maya bonesetting takes form not only via a difficult relationship with biomedicine but also through tense relationships between bonesetters. Maya bonesetters of different places often told me about specific clients who had been treated before by other bonesetters and how it had not gone well. They claimed that the other bonesetters did not really know how to treat injuries and that they themselves, basically, had to take over the cases. Bonesetters sometimes even seemed dismissive of other bonesetters, implying that they themselves had an ability that no one else had. As if to reinforce the point, most bonesetters attributed their own learning mostly to personal experience. Some reported that when they were kids, they saw a bonesetter work on one of their relatives, or that they even got treated themselves. But while this may have left an impression on them, they stressed that no one directly taught them the craft, that no one trained them. Crediting their work to their own life experience and intuition, bonesetters made no reference to any common store of knowledge that informed bonesetters as a whole. They would probably say that if Maya bonesetters practice in similar ways, it must be by coincidence. The bonesetters I met would likely play down the commonalities that I, as an outsider, see among bonesetters and that I built this book around.

When it comes to seeing commonalities, though, caution is warranted. While my depictions of Maya bonesetting might suggest that there is a generalized Maya bonesetting experience that can be distilled into neatly bounded variations, this is really not the case. The bonesetting practices I explore reflect how specific groups of Mayas work in specific times and places. Their practices and, just as important, how bonesetters justify them, play out in a late twentieth- to early twenty-first-century context in which unequal relations exist between Guatemala Mayas and nonindigenous Guatemalans. The bonesetters' methods for diagnosis and treatment are likewise affected by the kinds of diagnostic and treatment methods that institutional actors currently use, along with their technologies. That is, the bonesetters' work is driven both by what bonesetters personally find to be good practice and by what they believe clinicians do. They hear about what physicians do and they react to it, usually by criticizing practices such as casting and radiography. Bonesetters thus validate their practices by looking at their own results as well as by contrasting themselves with those medical actors who usually come from outside their communities and whose motives they find questionable. Doing this, they inhabit their place in what is probably a shifting continuum of bonesetting outlooks and techniques of which I caught only a glimpse.

The bottom line is that Maya bonesetting is historically situated. It is also uneven, with individual workers bringing varying degrees of experience, accepting different kinds of cases, and engaging in different ways with biomedicine. And as we will see, bonesetters are also working in different idioms that value distinct formative experiences and approaches, something that helps explain why some bonesetters are wary of other bonesetters. For instance, a bonesetter of a given group might disagree with the guiding idiom of the other group. Or he might argue that a bonesetter of group X is not complying with group X's own expectations. Bonesetters raise these concerns not because they want to discredit all other bonesetters, but because they believe their own methods are timeworn, proven, and worth keeping. To build a well-grounded picture of Maya bonesetting, then, I have had to approach many people, sift through many conversations, and mind how bonesetters were both alike and unlike each other. I have also focused heavily on the countryside, where most Guatemalan Mayas live and where the stakes are highest for them if they get injured.

Mayas and Bonesetting

Many Mayas practice bonesetting, and to learn about them I conducted research among two groups of highland Mayas in Guatemala. My work with Kaqchikel Mayas and Tz'utujiil Mayas brought me in contact with bonesetting traditions of different towns and regions, and this allowed me to see some important variations in their work. Through the ethnographic approach, I was able to observe how bonesetters engage in daily treatment practice, as well as how they talk about what they know. This approach also gave me a frame of reference for understanding bonesetting traditions outside the Maya area and those bonesetting practices that probably existed in the past. It should come as no surprise that bonesetting is needed and used virtually everywhere in Middle America. Many people who live there, after all, deal with the innumerable hardships tied to rural life and to the risks of an increasingly mechanized world. Given the similar hardships faced by people of other regions, it makes sense that manual medicine has long been practiced the world over (Ackerknecht 1947; Agarwal and Agarwal 2010; Clark 1937). Bodies are everywhere susceptible to injury, and the injured try to find treatment options that are accessible, affordable, and effective (Majno 1975; Oths and Hinojosa 2004).

Since many people in Guatemala today work in manual medicine, at times working with bones and at other times not, I will clarify that I follow Brad Huber and Robert Anderson's use of the term "bonesetter": "A bonesetter is someone who, in addition to massage, moves bones as a form of medical treatment. The most obvious association customarily made for the term is that a bonesetter reduces (sets) fractures. Less obvious is the fact that a bonesetter may also induce motion in painful or impaired joints" (1996:31). Those individuals I call bonesetters engage in these activities, though they handle fractures less often than they do other injuries. The reduction of fractures, in fact, constitutes but one manual medicine specialty among many in Middle America. Manual medicine workers in the region focus primarily on massaging muscle and other soft tissue; these are the parts of the body people most often injure. My interactions with bonesetters made this clear. What also became clear is that, had I not spent the time that I did (see below) with the bonesetters, I might not have learned much about them. To this day, there exists little published research about bonesetting in this region.

Only a few ethnographic works have dealt with bonesetting in modern Middle American groups. What we currently know about Maya bonesetters can be found in works by Hinojosa (2002, 2004b, 2004c), Hugo Icú Perén (1990), Clarence Edward McMahon (1994), Benjamin Paul (1976), and Paul and Clancy E. McMahon (2001), who each conducted research specifically on bonesetters. Numerous other researchers refer to Maya bonesetters, but usually in the process of listing the different health specialists found in native communities. Still, these works and others like them have gone a long way toward reaffirming that bonesetters are common in the places where Mayas live.[1] And while they are also common outside of the Maya area, there, too, their activities have remained underreported. Our knowledge of bonesetting in non-Maya areas of Mexico comes largely from the researchers Paolo Femia (1992), Huber and Anderson (1996), Xavier Lozoya Legorreta et al. (1988), and a few others.[2] Some researchers have focused on therapeutic massage specialists working in Mexico (R. Anderson 1987; McClain 1976) and, in doing so, have highlighted the continuities that exist between the work of *sobadores* (folk massagers) and the work of curers who actively manipulate bones. These scholars and others who have worked among a variety of cultural groups in Mexico have added to the picture of bonesetting as it exists over a wide area. Other recent bonesetting traditions are known to us from lower Central America (Peterson 1994), the Andes (Oths 2002, 2004; Salvador Hernández 2011), and the Amazon basin (*Science News Letter* 1938), but information on bonesetting in these areas is also lacking.

The relatively few studies of bonesetting practices in the Americas contrast with the many examples of research on bonesetters from other parts of the world. Many of these works focus on places with long histories of therapeutic massage and bonesetting, including Africa,[3] Asia,[4] the Middle East,[5] and Europe.[6] But while there exists more published research about bonesetting in these places than in the Americas, writings about bonesetting outside the Western Hemisphere have often been very critical of the practice, much of this research having been carried out by biomedical practitioners, who have shown a low regard for bonesetting to begin with. Many of their publications focus disproportionately upon failed cases of traditional bonesetting, particularly those with crippling outcomes (Burford et al. 2007:367–369). This research, moreover, scrutinizes bonesetting practices in terms of institutional medical precepts that did not actually emerge until long after the bonesetting traditions had taken shape. In this way these researchers hold bonesetters to rather high clinical standards, even though bonesetters developed largely outside clinical contexts. Seeing bonesetting through a strictly medical lens presents many problems, some of which I will explore later in this book.

When researchers have turned their attention to bonesetters in Guatemala and Mexico, however, their approach has not carried the same tone of disapproval, or even reproach, that often pervades research done outside the Americas. By and large, research on Mesoamerican bonesetting has focused on how bonesetters do their work and what tools they use. It shows how their vocations connect with rural life, with the landscape, and with the material resources at hand, many of which seem to change every few years. The research also explores how physicians routinely cast bonesetters as unqualified and potentially dangerous. And while these works provide only a partial portrait of bonesetting, they still confirm that bonesetters have long been important to people in the region, despite their detractors. This importance relates directly to the places featured in this book.

A Few Words on Methods

I first heard about Maya bonesetters when getting to know residents of San Juan Comalapa, a Kaqchikel community in the central Guatemalan highlands. Comalapans told me that when local people got injured—whether in the fields, at home, or on the road—they would go visit some local curers who could treat injuries using only their hands. This was in 1992, when I was doing my early graduate work and when I was trying to learn about Maya healers. With a lot of curiosity on my part, and with the help of two Kaqchikel Maya families, I was able to locate and meet three bonesetters. I began interviewing these men and interacting with them as much as I could, and thanks to them I made some good inroads into the local meanings of bonesetting. But before long, my dissertation work took center stage and my research went in a different direction. My work on Maya bonesetting would have to wait.

During one of the years in which I was doing my doctoral fieldwork, 1995, I met two additional bonesetters. One was Tonia, whom I was able to meet only briefly. The other was Eduardo, whom I spoke with in Panabajal, one of Comalapa's larger satellite villages, where he lived.[7] When I resumed my research on bonesetters in 1998, I ventured beyond Comalapa to the towns of San Pedro La Laguna and San Juan La Laguna, two communities straddling Lake Atitlán. I had learned that there were numerous bonesetters living and working there (B. Paul 1976). With a friend's help, I started meeting Maya bonesetters in these towns and so brought three male bonesetters from San Pedro La Laguna into my study. That same year (1998) I was also able to meet two female bonesetters from San Pedro La Laguna, one of whom was the daughter of a male bonesetter I had met earlier. As with the bone specialists from Comalapa, I spent as much time as I could listening to the San Pedro La Laguna bonesetters and observing their work. When I returned the following year, in 1999, I tracked down two additional male bonesetters in San Juan La Laguna whom I had been referred to earlier.

In the meantime, I lived in Comalapa for part of each field season, so I made it a point to continue visiting with the bonesetters I knew there and to ask about other ones. This allowed me to meet three local bonesetters I had not crossed paths with before, two in 2000 and one in 2001. In the latter year, during a visit to San Juan La Laguna, I also met with the daughter of a local bonesetter, who was a practicing bonesetter herself. This presaged my meeting in 2002 with the son of a San Pedro La Laguna bonesetter, who had begun practicing bonesetting in the wake of his father's recent death. In 2002 I also located an additional female bonesetter in San Pedro La Laguna and spoke with her about her work.

My interaction with the bonesetters took place mainly in their homes, where they perform most of their treatments. I learned about their work by speaking with them in both unstructured and semistructured ways and sometimes by watching them treat people. When bonesetters treated someone in my presence, they usually worked quietly, pausing to speak with the client, then turning to explain to me what their hands were doing and what their hands had found. At times I spoke with the bonesetters' clients, both those I met at treatment encounters and others I met in the course of town life, especially in Comalapa. They often told me how they were doing since they had been treated by the bonesetters; they also told me what they thought about different bonesetters. But the bonesetters themselves were my most important teachers. Welcoming me into their homes and shops, they were more than gracious with their time, and very patient with my questions. I was lucky to find them at home when I did because, as people who divide their time between regular work and bonesetting, at any given hour they were just as likely to be away treating someone or working in their fields as they were to be treating someone at home. The busiest of bonesetters might spend more time away from home than under his or her own roof, but I met only one person such as this (in San Pedro La Laguna), and he, too, attended to his own fields when he was home. As I determined the best times to reach individual bonesetters, it became clearer that not only did their daily work vary enormously, but they were especially busy on certain days, for example, market days. More people would arrive on those days in Comalapa, for example, and might take the opportunity to visit a bonesetter. Over time, though, as I met with bonesetters, I got to know some of them better than others, and the former naturally left a deeper imprint on my work. Nevertheless, even the short interactions I had with some bonesetters helped to answer some of my questions and contributed to my thinking. To this day their generosity and calm demeanor still shape the way I view their craft.[8]

In the time I spent with Comalapa bonesetters, I witnessed about twelve treatments, plus received one. Local bonesetters also told me about around forty-eight cases they had handled, describing some in more detail than others. In San Pedro La Laguna and San Juan La Laguna, meanwhile, I saw about eight treatment encounters, plus another twenty-eight treatments that a San Pedro La Laguna bonesetter performed in nearby Santiago Atitlán. Bonesetters in San Pedro La Laguna and San Juan La Laguna also told me about twenty-three of their clients and how they treated them. In Comalapa, San Pedro La Laguna, and San Juan La Laguna, I also met an untold number of people who had been treated by bonesetters at least once in their lives.

To round out my learning about Maya bonesetters, I also reached out to and spoke with nine physicians. Six of them lived and worked in Comalapa, including one who was the attending physician at the Comalapa Health Center. Another physician was from Comalapa but oversaw the community health organization Asociación de Servicios Comunitarios de Salud (ASECSA), located in Comalapa's department capital, Chimaltenango, where I also interviewed one of the organization's nonphysician administrators. In San Pedro La Laguna, meanwhile, I spoke with the attending physician at the local health center, as well as with other personnel there. To this sample I added a physician working in Panajachel, the largest town and traffic hub on the shore of Lake Atitlán, through which many injured people pass en route to either San Pedro La Laguna or the department capital, Sololá. Drawing from their backgrounds in public and private practice, the physicians gave me their appraisals of bonesetters. They also shared with me their abiding concerns for people who get injured, people who, in their view, may or may not be treated adequately by bonesetters. And though only two of the nine physicians offered even a tempered endorsement of what bonesetters do, they clearly knew the long odds bonesetters faced. They knew how people took all kinds of injuries to bonesetters, injuries that might challenge even the skills of clinicians who practice in rural areas. In the end, though, and despite their many misgivings about bonesetters, the physicians helped me to better situate the bonesetters' work within the larger landscape of health-care providers.

Interacting with these physicians, organizational staffers, bonesetters, and everyday people, I was left with the impression that manual medicine affects people of many backgrounds in one way or another. It might vex the assumptions of one group (physicians), define the approach of another (bonesetters), and bring relief to yet another (clients). Amidst these interactions, something else came to stand out about manual medicine: the bulk of bonesetting seems to be in the hands of men, a situation not unique to the communities in this study.

Bonesetting and Gender

In twentieth-century Mesoamerican communities, bonesetting appears to have been mainly the province of men (Huber and Anderson 1996; Rodríguez Rouanet 1969:55; Tedlock 1992:74; Wisdom 1940:355).[9] There may be several reasons for this: Many occupational factors connect rural people (Berlin and Berlin 1996:58), and men in particular (Harvey 2013:80–81), with traumatic injury. The heaviest work in rural communities—such as subsistence agriculture, lumbering, construction, transportation, and large-animal handling—tends to be carried out by males, placing them at high risk for severe work injuries. In a study of Kaqchikel Maya bonesetters, most of the bonesetters' clients were found to be males under age thirty-four, highlighting this sector as the most vulnerable to musculoskeletal injury (Icú Perén 1990:64). Accordingly, Marianna Appel Kunow (2003:51) notes that in the Yucatec Maya community she studied, "male [bonesetter] patients may outnumber female patients simply because men's work in the *milpa* renders them more susceptible to . . . injuries." Over the course of their lives, Maya men spend many of their working hours in the fields and forests, and many can recount cases of injuries they have experienced or witnessed there. In addition, soccer fields have become prime injury grounds, and, here again, younger men have the bruises, sprains, and dislocations to prove it. These factors might help account for the greater exposure of men to traumatic injury, but the propensity of men to work in bonesetting is more difficult to explain.

Part of the answer may lie in men's proximity to accident sites. Men injured in the hills must rely on those around them, usually other men, for immediate help. Certain men are therefore forced to deal with difficult injury cases as best as they can on the spot. In doing this, they might develop a reputation for having successfully handled emergencies, and, gradually, more cases are brought to them. Men might also be favored as bonesetters because of the strength needed to lift and pull the heavier limbs of adults. As the Comalapan bonesetter Lupito remarks, "In order to treat, some strength is needed, also, especially if you're dealing with the knee . . . sometimes strength is needed." Comments by an elderly female bonesetter in Comalapa,[10] and by another female bonesetter in San Pedro La Laguna, echo this view (B. Paul 1976:77). However, bonesetters also point out that it takes more than sheer strength to perform bonesetting: it takes focused moves. A Tz'utujiil bonesetter of San Pedro La Laguna exemplifies this when he tells me about moving bones: "It doesn't have anything to do with strength; you have to do it gently." So while some physical strength is required of bonesetters, extreme strength is not, for we know that elderly men and women can be effective bonesetters (Douglas 1969:135). Maya women, furthermore, have repeatedly demonstrated great manual dexterity in midwifery (Cosminsky 2016; Hinojosa 2004a). To move bones, though, one does have to be *valiente* (courageous) (Huber and Anderson 1996:27). The Comalapan bonesetter Paulino says it takes *valor* (nerve, courage) to be able to witness pain and to fix bones. The nature of the work demands it.

In light of how men in Mesoamerica carry out some of the most hazardous work and how they are likely to be around when injury happens, Kunow's (2003:46) assertion that the work of bonesetters "appears to be an exclusively male domain" can be better contextualized. Her view also concurs with the findings of Icú Perén (1990:42), who noticed the preponderance of male bonesetters in Comalapa when he wrote about local bonesetters for his medical thesis. But while male bonesetters likely outnumber female ones in the region, there are still many female bonesetters. The fact remains that by not including more females in this study, and by not reaching the conversational ease with them that I did with males, I limited the scope of this book. Although these pages can claim much information about the cultural meanings of bonesetting, it probably lacks insights about female bonesetters. And while I cannot undo this omission here, I can restate what female bonesetters have told me about themselves and about other female bonesetters and hope that it closes the knowledge gap a little. Later research will be needed to expand on how many female bonesetters, who by their own report tend to work with other women and with children, actually handle a wide range of injury cases (Car et al. 2005: 80; McMahon 1994).

The Setting

Getting to meet Maya bonesetters was rewarding in itself, but I also got to see the distinct spaces where the two main groups of bonesetters worked. Strong contrasts among the towns became apparent early on. One of the first things I noticed was how relatively isolated Comalapa was compared with the towns of San Pedro La Laguna and San Juan La Laguna. Comalapa is located in mountainous terrain, and during the bulk of the time I spent there it was reachable only by an unreliable, winding dirt road that connected it to a town on the Inter-American Highway. It was thus less likely to be visited by casual travelers than were the towns of San Pedro La Laguna and San Juan La Laguna, which are close neighbors on the sloping shore of highland Lake Atitlán. One effect of this is that a large number of foreign tourists inhabit the streets, restaurants, and hotels of San Pedro La Laguna and, to a lesser degree, San Juan La Laguna. This accessibility makes for a striking mixture of sounds, languages, and people in the two lakeside towns of a kind seldom seen in Comalapa.

The three towns differ in other ways as well. Whereas Comalapa is home to Kaqchikel Mayas, the native inhabitants of San Pedro La Laguna and San Juan La Laguna are Tz'utujiil Mayas. Kaqchikel and Tz'utujiil speakers can understand much of each other's languages, but when meeting in markets or buses they will often switch to Spanish. As is today usually the case with inhabitants of rural communities in Guatemala, most people of Comalapa, San Pedro La Laguna, and San Juan La Laguna either can speak Spanish or can function in it. Of those who speak only Spanish, most are culturally Ladino, Guatemalans who do not personally identify with any Maya culture. Although people considered Ladinos tend to live in large cities and in the urban core of rural communities, in those rural areas Ladinos are usually dwarfed in number by the local indigenous population. This is certainly the case in Comalapa, where a recent population census found that over 79 percent of its population is indigenous, though the actual proportion of the population that is Kaqchikel Maya is likely much higher.[11] The proportion of indigenous population in San Pedro La Laguna and in San Juan La Laguna is probably nearly as high as Comalapa's.

One last area of difference has to do with the ways that bonesetters approach their work in Comalapa versus in the lakeside towns. In Comalapa, Mayas who practice bonesetting take a highly practical and pragmatic approach. They learn their skills in physical ways, and they apply them physically to obtain physical results. Bonesetters of San Pedro La Laguna and San Juan La Laguna, meanwhile, also practice physical manipulation to get physical results, but they avowedly do their work in the context of having been divinely chosen for it, and they use revealed objects to diagnose and treat. Their shared bonesetting tradition is strikingly different from that of Comalapa's and, I venture, from most other bonesetting traditions of Mesoamerica. I will discuss the main features of these two types of bonesetting, empirical and sacred, in chapters 2 and 3.

This book thus explores the experiences and work of bonesetters in these two very dissimilar communities, broadly speaking. I bring in the perspectives of eighteen Maya bonesetters I had the privilege of meeting, only several of whom are still alive today. By interacting with them over the years, watching them work in their homes, or accompanying them on house calls, I have come to see how individual bonesetters value different aspects of their work, as well as how their respective communities appreciate them. Local people express a real need for them because there is a real need for them. Just as few rural indigenous people express comfort about going to clinicians for help with their pregnancies and deliveries, few also express a preference for the physician over the bonesetter when injuries happen. Physicians make this vividly clear when they describe how local people do not put clinicians at the top of their caregiver list when they need help with infirmity or injury. Consider what physicians in Comalapa say about bonesetters and other curers: Dr. Sucuc remarks that "people never go first with the doctor"; they go to either local healers or the pharmacy first. Dr. Icú Perén similarly relates that sick people go first to the curer, then to the pharmacy, then to a service institution, for instance, the Health Center, and last to a private physician. This pattern of help-seeking is apparent in the rural area, says another clinician, Dr. Serech. He explains that people in rural areas prefer treating themselves first with curers, "but as a final alternative they go with [a physician]." Taking such behaviors into account, Dr. Suárez feels convinced, as he puts it, "the people have more faith in them [bonesetters] than in us [doctors]."

As much as these remarks might suggest that rural people have little use for physicians, this is emphatically not the case. However, though rural Guatemalans do seek out and use physicians, they also make their health decisions in living contexts that many feel are outside of the expertise of clinicians. For this reason, most rural Mayas take their pregnant family members to midwives and take their injured relatives to bone-setters. Such can be the gravity and frequency of their injuries, in fact, that Mayas also seek help from non-Maya bonesetters at times.[12] These patterns will likely continue because if national health data suggest anything about the prevalence of injury in Guatemala, it is that life in Guatemala, especially in rural areas, is not becoming any easier.

The Injury Landscape of Guatemala

We see this most clearly in the way that accidents abound in both work-spaces and roadways. Whether people are working at home, which is a primary workspace throughout Guatemala and particularly for women in the rural areas, or are using roads and highways, they face a recurrent risk of injury. While the home space may not conjure images of high-risk activities, the many burns and falls that occur there indicate otherwise, to say nothing of the intentional injuries stemming from violence between partners. So problematic have falls in general become that, according to 2014 World Health Organization (WHO) records, falls are the forty-eighth leading cause of death in Guatemala.[13] And while both men and women are affected by falls, most of the women I saw treated by bonesetters, and whom bonesetters spoke of as clients, had been injured by falls on roads and steps. This record suggests that the home and its associated spaces—markets, washbasins, and the like—present real risks for women. With changes to roadways, moreover, entirely new risks are affecting wider circles of Guatemalans.

In recent decades, more Guatemalan roadways have been leveled and paved. And while this has led to easier transportation between communities, it has also led to vehicles moving at higher speeds. This was certainly the case when the dirt road connecting Comalapa with the town on the Inter-American Highway, Zaragoza, had its asphalting completed in the late 1990s. Travel time between the two towns diminished, but many Comalapans worried about how fast the intercity buses now drove, fearful they might fall victim to the crashes that they increasingly heard about. Many passengers, including me, had probably been in buses on other high-speed, rain-slicked highways, with a driver holding the steering wheel in one hand and a cellphone in the other. Worsening this picture is the buses' practice of racing each other down asphalted highways to pick up passengers standing on the roadside. For Comalapans, the thought of local bus drivers rushing through the blind mountain curves certainly did not inspire confidence in road safety.

Taken together, these conditions have given rise to many vehicular injuries and deaths. In fact, road traffic accidents have become the seventeenth leading cause of death in Guatemala.[14] A big part of the problem is the nonseparation of space between those who drive trucks, cars, motorcycles, or bicycles. Another part centers on the many people who hitchhike, ride unprotected in the back of trucks and on top of buses, and rarely use seatbelts when riding in an automobile. The high rate of traffic fatalities confirms the WHO observation that Guatemala is witnessing more injuries than ever before, especially "due to external causes such as road traffic or violence."[15] In general, the most vulnerable road users, pedestrians, shoulder an especially high burden of injury (Peden et al. 2004:41). This is due to high levels of foot traffic near already dangerous roadways and to poor crossing infrastructure.

Guatemalans know that injury is a fact of life, but this really stands out when considering how their vulnerability to a broad range of injuries has been worsening over the years and disfavors men in particular. Findings from 2002, 2004, and 2008 tell us a lot. Government records from 2002, for instance, report that in over 80 percent of rural Maya homes in which a member has an incapacity of an upper or lower extremity, the person with the incapacity is male.[16] WHO data from two years later explain more about this connection between males and injuries, showing that in 2004, over four times as many men as women died from an injury, five times as many men as women died from road traffic accidents, twice as many men as women died from falls, almost three times as many men as women died from "other unintentional injuries," and seven times as many men as women died from "intentional injuries," for example, violent acts.[17] WHO data from 2008 initially suggest a continuation of the male vulnerability trend: the proportion of men dying from injury is high and increasing; the proportion of men and women dying from falls is increasing; and the proportion of men dying from "other unintentional injuries" remains at the level reported earlier, higher than for women.[18] Bear in mind, though, that these data are from cases reported to health and legal authorities, so they are likely underestimates.

These data reflect the pattern of male susceptibility to injury discussed earlier, but they also show that there is more to the picture, that men are not the only ones experiencing harm. Data from different sources point to vectors of change directly affecting women. For one, the data signal alarming changes with respect to road traffic accidents, with the proportion of women killed on the increase by 2008.[19] The findings do not say whether this is due to greater mixed road use and increased passenger loads, but it is clear that injury remains an increasingly significant cause of death for women, and this trend shows no signs of abating. Given the fact that more women than before work outside the home, and that jobs require more roadway travel than before, we should be mindful of Lewis Zirkle's (2008: 2443) finding that road traffic accidents are a "disease of emerging prosperity." As people commute to work more, they spend much more time on the road. They might even spend their earnings on obtaining a vehicle of their own, one that will become the family vehicle and that will most likely increase the injury vulnerability of the entire household.

The ways in which exposure to injury is changing in Guatemala speak to how, in the words of a WHO study, "health-care challenges are greater in regions with predominantly indigenous, rural and poor populations."[20] Simply being from a "disadvantaged socioeconomic group(s) or living in poorer areas" places one at greater risk of being injured or killed in traffic, as Margie Peden et al. (2004:46) have argued. Exposure to traffic risks can thus be seen as an expression of how disproportionately heavy the workload of indigenous people in rural areas is, as well as of the greater work demands being placed on women.

But even more troubling is the evidence that women are being injured without ever leaving the home, and that much of this is due to domestic violence. The proportion of women dying from "intentional injuries" is growing, according to a 2008 WHO report.[21] Official Guatemalan statistics further show that in 2008, there were nearly ten times as many reported Maya female victims of domestic violence as there were Maya male victims.[22] The same document reports, moreover, that Maya women are most vulnerable to *violencia intrafamiliar* between the ages of twenty and twenty-nine (Maya men, meanwhile, are reportedly most active and aggressive between the ages of twenty-five and thirty-four). Increasing levels of violence in the home might also point to heightened levels of economic stress and to an environment of legal impunity for abusers. This lack of accountability against aggressors complicates an already vulnerable situation for Guatemalan women, with the unresponsive legal system discouraging women from even going to the authorities for help (Walsh and Menjívar 2016).

The growing victimization of women that injury records reflect is worrisome in itself, but the systemic underreporting of these injuries is equally troubling. Having only limited data makes it hard to determine just how much domestic violence is happening in Maya homes, and how much is being concealed. The uncertainty about how much abuse is happening is partly due to (an overreliance on) government facilities as responsible parties for reporting abuse, something in turn complicated by the limited availability of medical facilities in rural areas.[23] The underreporting of injuries in general to local clinicians, and the subsequent underreporting by these individuals to state health officials, adds to the vulnerability picture of Mayas and other rural people, and reminds us to accept official health figures with caution.

Health Center Records and Partial Glimpses of the Local

Despite the previously listed difficulties, a look at some recent records from community health centers can still be revealing. For example, it can show how current record-keeping practices supply at best a sketchy picture of how many community members suffer injuries. It can also offer a look at the kinds of injuries people bring to local health authorities. The information supplied by official health centers in San Juan Comalapa and San Pedro La Laguna provides a useful lens into injury experience at the local level, even if the data each center provides differ significantly.

To identify how many people have come to each health center with injuries in recent years, as well as to identify the sex of each patient, personnel at each center searched their computer records for patients whose diagnoses include *traumatismo* or *politraumatismo*. These terms generally mean "injury" and "multiple injuries" due to physical impacts, and may or may not include injuries that involve lacerations. Because I am most interested in identifying injuries caused by falls, accidents, and blows and that do not involve open wounds, the center personnel narrowed their searches as much as possible to find these cases. Completing its search, the Comalapa Health Center then provided me with listed aggregated numbers of users, male and female, who were diagnosed with a traumatismo or politraumatismo each year from 2005 to 2015 and in 2017. The San Pedro La Laguna Health Center, meanwhile, provided tables containing information about individual deidentified patients whose diagnoses included any *traumatismo*. The tables encompass the years 2011 to 2017 and include the sex of each patient as well as a brief diagnostic summary. Although each center provides data in discrete formats, each body of data delivers revealing insights into the local occurrence of injury and, equally important, into the reporting of injury.

Reviewing the 2,579 cases of traumatismo and politraumatismo reported in Comalapa in the years 2005 to 2015 and 2017, for instance, shows one immediately apparent trend. In the years for which records are available, there are generally increasing numbers of reported nonspecific injuries of both men and women in the municipality. This initially suggests a growing overall susceptibility to injury in the area, but other factors could be at work. The health center's attending physician, Dr. Sotz', for one, attributes much of the general growth in numbers to the fact that, in 2009, the health center began to operate twenty-four hours a day, every day; it was previously open from 8:00 a.m. to 4:00 p.m. from Monday to Friday. With the change to round-the-clock hours and especially weekend availability, he stresses, many more people have been coming to the center. Many of these individuals might have otherwise gone to the department capital for care, or they might have not sought care at all, but it is not possible to tell. At any rate, the number of people reporting injuries to the center in 2009 (n = 203), when it began to function twenty-four hours a day, climbed 52.6 percent over the previous year's number (n = 133), when the center had limited operating hours. The numbers of people reporting injuries continued a steady climb in the years that followed, reaching 538 cases in 2015 and 413 cases in 2017, the last years on record.

A few points should be raised about these figures, however. Since traumatismo and politraumatismo are categories of nonspecific injury that may or may not include lacerations, there are likely many other cases of injuries (e.g., filed under *lesionados* and *accidentados*) taken to the health center but not included here, in addition to those that go completely unreported. This differential diagnostic coding may suppress the numbers of people who appear to have brought traumatic injuries to the health center. As it now stands, in eleven of the twelve years between 2005 and 2017 (excluding 2016, during which records were not recorded properly, says Dr. Sotz'), males reported more injuries than did females. And while this would be in keeping with the high risks attendant to the typical arenas of male work, it is still necessary to question whether injuries suffered by women, especially those that might reflect poorly on families, are being withheld from the health center. It is most telling, then, that the attending physician says that the health center numbers represent fewer than half of all the local people who get injured. Dr. Sotz' remarks, "In reality there are very few" who come compared with the likely numbers of people who suffer injuries in the municipality. He also admits that his records contain inadequate information about people who bring serious injuries to the health center. This is because when persons with possible fractures arrive, the center immediately sends them to have radiographs taken in Chimaltenango, the department capital. In the end, because the health center lacks the capacity to treat people, as Dr. Sotz' observes, it does not treat severe injuries.

Following a search for reported traumatismo cases at the San Pedro La Laguna Health Center, meanwhile, I found another distinct local picture emerging. Personnel at the center identified 229 cases containing a traumatismo diagnosis between 2011 and 2017, but while the number of reported injury cases there in 2011 (n = 11) was far surpassed by the number of injury cases later reported in 2017 (n = 91), the intervening years do not show as steady a climb in injury numbers as we see in Comalapa. There is more fluctuation in the number of injury cases reported every year in San Pedro La Laguna. Neither do we see a clear pattern of males or females reporting more injuries in the lakeside community, with males reporting more injuries in four of the seven years covered and females reporting more injuries in three of those years. And even though the San Pedro La Laguna Health Center, like its Comalapa counterpart, began operating around the clock and seven days a week in 2009, San Pedro La Laguna center personnel do not connect an immediate change in usership to that event.

What patterns do emerge from the health center figures, however, are striking. For example, of the 229 injury cases located by health center personnel, only about half (n = 111) name an injured body part, and of these cases, 66.7 percent (n = 74) refer to the head or to a part of the face as the injured area. This finding suggests that when people bring to the health center injuries that can be readily associated with specific parts of the body, two-thirds of the time those body parts are the head and face, areas of the body that local bonesetters do not usually work with. Moreover, only 6.5 percent (n = 15) of all traumatismo cases name an affected limb or joint in a limb, or refer to "tendons and muscles"—all parts of the body that bonesetters *do* typically work with. Taken together, this means that injured people come to the health center for injuries that bonesetters *do not* usually treat (e.g., of the head) and that they only rarely take non-life-threatening injuries of the extremities (e.g., arms and legs) to the health center. The likelihood that health center clinicians will see injury cases thus depends on what part of the body is injured: if it is a body part that bonesetters usually treat, the data suggest that the clinicians are less likely to see it. The health center is not in a position to see or document these kinds of cases in the way it might document cases brought to the center.

As it turns out, even the injury cases that this health center documents run short on detail. Some 85.2 percent of all reported injury cases (n = 195), for example, denote "nonspecific" in some way, with respect to either which body part was affected or the degree to which it was affected. Unfortunately, this record-keeping practice renders nearly invisible these most salient features of injury cases, even if it simplifies data coding at the point of contact with the patient. When I describe how the San Pedro La Laguna Health Center records frequently use the term *no especificado* to Dr. Hugo Icú Perén, director of ASECSA in Chimaltenango, he tells me something rather surprising. When health center physicians examine patients, "tratan de colocar el diagnóstico menos compromedor para ellos" (they try to assign a diagnosis that is the least binding for them). According to him, recorded decisions about cases have as much to do with a desire to avoid committing to a specific diagnosis as they do with an interest in brevity. Physicians accept this diagnostic ambiguity about traumatismos in part because, as they often tell me, they cannot get exact information about possible fractures or dislocations without an X-ray, and preferring to err on the side of caution, they send their patients to the nearest X-ray facility. Injured people in San Pedro La Laguna might thus be sent to get X-rays in the national hospital located in the department capital, Sololá, but if they go, their cases will not normally be further documented in the San Pedro La Laguna Health Center computer system. Information about injuries that originate in the community, then, remains patchy. However, people do seem to be taking injuries of their arms and legs to people other than health center clinicians, and health center clinicians seem to rely on out-of-town technology to deal with those severe cases that they can only tentatively diagnose.

For all they reveal about who reports injuries to the two health centers, what may be most telling about these health center figures is how they offer just a glimpse of local injury experience. The information the centers can capture is limited because, from the outset, they are only intended to cover most, but not all, of their respective populations. In Comalapa, for example, Dr. Sotz' says the Centro de Salud covers only 60 percent of the population, leaving the other 40 percent to be covered by the Guatemalan Social Security Institute, private physicians, and out-of-town hospitals. Echoing what senior personnel at the San Pedro La Laguna Health Center say, he reports that the injured people they do receive, moreover, are few in number and that their injuries usually come from work mishaps, not vehicular accidents. A further limit of the records is how they do not note how many of their users they sent for care elsewhere, or how many users came after initially receiving treatment elsewhere. In both places, in fact, the health center records do not account for injury cases of people who go elsewhere to get a final diagnosis, a notable lacuna in the data because the centers normally outsource their diagnoses for severe trauma cases.[24]

In terms of local center users, men seem more prone to suffering injury, or at least to reporting injury, in the two communities, even if this raises doubts about whether something might be suppressing women's injury numbers. The vulnerability of women to injury remains an open question. What information exists, in San Pedro La Laguna at least, suggests that the kinds of injury taken to the health center might not have been taken to Maya bonesetters anyway. Still, relatively few local people bring their injuries to the health centers, which has probably led to systemic under-reporting and underrecording of injury cases. Incomplete health data may be part of the reason trauma or lesions do not appear among, or connected to, the top twenty leading causes of mortality in Comalapa, San Pedro La Laguna, or San Juan La Laguna, according to a government health report covering the years 2012 to 2016.[25] The same report also excludes trauma or lesions from its listing of the top few causes of morbidity in these com-munities during the same time period.[26] At the local level and in clini-cal spaces, it seems that information about traumatismo and politrauma-tismo cases remains uneven and perhaps suggests that health centers are stressing other priorities.

Health Centers, Priorities, and Nascent Partnerings

Health centers do emphasize services connected to the well-being of mothers and children, typically within a framework of upgrading over-all community health. And the degree to which health centers prioritize maternal-infant health and attendant areas such as disease prevention and nutrition also affects the centers' approach to community outreach. In line with their stated health objectives, health centers have thus taken a strong interest in developing ties with community midwives. This strategy has typically taken the form of identifying practicing midwives, "invit-ing" them to training sessions (*capacitaciones*), issuing them a certifica-tion (*carnet*), mandating that they change their practices to conform to health center requirements, and thereafter requiring them to return for follow-up courses. In the decades since launching this model of commu-nity health intervention, health centers have identified and licensed thou-sands of practicing Maya midwives, and have kept lists of midwives who are allowed to practice under this system.[27]

However many midwives have been allowed to work through this pro-gram, the overall scheme has proven highly problematic for them. As re-searchers have shown, the training to which midwives have had to submit shows a disconnect between the "official" knowledge that health center trainers purvey and what midwives know from practice (Berry 2006:1962; Cosminsky 2016:208, 216, 225). The power asymmetry inherent in these arrangements intensifies long-standing inequalities between health center staff, usually of non-Maya background, and Maya midwives (Chary et al. 2013). Increasing numbers of Maya midwives have also reported discrimination and mistreatment by health center and hospital personnel in accounts conveyed through national media (Julajuj 2017a; Sánchez 2017). At this point, however, the Ministry of Public Health and Social Assistance (shortened to Ministry of Public Health in this book) seems set on continuing to train midwives with an aim to improving pregnancy outcomes, particularly within a renewed framework of care launched following the 1996 Peace Accords (Maupin 2008). The health centers continue to see midwives as essential adjuncts to care, even if their relations with them remain deeply strained. For all their interest in these healers, health centers have not shown an equally high interest in other kinds of healers. Bonesetters are conspicuously absent from their formulations for creating community health partnerships. Why health centers have not reached out to Maya bonesetters, or seriously thought about them as potential partners, speaks to unique aspects of the bonesetters' work. The health centers' position on bonesetters evidently derives as much from what midwives and bonesetters actually handle as from the different ways that these practitioners engage with Guatemala's legal landscape. And of these practitioners, only midwives, for legal reasons discussed in the next paragraph, have seemed appealing in any way to the health system. The result is that midwives have been drawn into routinized relationships with health centers, relationships that are not currently possible for bonesetters.

Midwives appear more amenable to working with the health system than bonesetters do for a number of reasons. Preeminent among these is that pregnancy and childbirth differ a great deal from physical injury. Pregnancy has a beginning, a middle, and an end, and generally has a clear resolution. Further, the pregnancy and birth process ends with a legal document of birth, an *acta de nacimiento*. Childbirth affects population, schools, and down-the-road infrastructure and health spending, so there is a political stake in having it monitored and recorded. Injury, meanwhile, has neither pregnancy's clear progression (except usually a beginning) nor a legally binding outcome, for example, a certificate of health. Bonesetting, then, is not bound to a bureaucratic structure like the work of midwives is. This probably deflects official state interest away from bonesetting.

Of the other structural reasons that have drawn midwives into the health system, the main one is that for several decades (and particularly since the 1976 earthquake) the Ministry of Public Health has, as mentioned earlier, required practicing midwives to submit to formal training and certifications. After receiving their initial training, midwives are supposed to attend later training sessions, even if this takes them out of town at their own expense. In addition, they must keep records of their maternity clients on file with the health center, recommend difficult cases to physicians, and initiate the paperwork for each birth.[28] Moreover, at the health center's behest, registered midwives must also identify and reach out to other practicing midwives who have not yet registered with the health center. If these "invited" midwives do not present themselves to the health center, they are considered to be working extralegally. From the ministry's point of view, midwives should work in line with the health center's programs, as well as enforce its rules, turning midwives into purveyors of the government's policies. Whenever there is a vaccination campaign, for instance; a concern about dengue, cholera, or other diseases; or a program to encourage birth-spacing (i.e., the Asociación Pro-Familia [APROFAM]), midwives have been tasked as the health center's standard-bearers. This is because they can reach into far more homes than health center personnel can. In short, midwifery in Guatemala today, which is largely in the hands of Maya women, is heavily defined and constrained by functionaries of the Ministry of Public Health through health centers.

Bonesetters, meanwhile, work in an arena that is less officially tied into what the health structure considers the most revealing metrics of health: birth, perinatal mortality, infant mortality, child mortality, maternal mortality, prevalent forms of morbidity, leading causes of mortality, and, increasingly, chronic diseases with high morbidity and mortality outcomes. And though the state has shown interest in documenting some raw numbers of traumatic injury cases per annum, as I discussed in an earlier section, these cases have generally gone underreported. When these cases are reported, moreover, no distinction is made between those that are brought directly to health center personnel and those that might have been treated first by a bonesetter. As a result, not as much is known about the rates of traumatic injury as about other metrics of health more closely tied to midwifery. With the health problems that bonesetters deal with accorded a lower priority, the work of bonesetters assumes an ever lower profile.

In the end, midwives and bonesetters are not exactly commensurate in terms of their historical possibilities for integration into, or compatibility with, the health system, something that tracks back to what their hands actually handle. Their possibilities for integration are likely also affected by how the health centers' priorities include not just shaping certain measurable health outcomes but also shaping certain local people into helpful partners. Up until now midwives have been accorded more possibilities in this regard, especially since their work already sits astride bureaucratic processes of birth registry, which explains in large measure why midwives have well surpassed bonesetters in their degree of official inclusion in health systems. It also suggests why the bonesetters' degree of integration into health systems has been very uneven on a global scale: when it comes to recognizing and partnering with bonesetters, medical authorities are not of one mind (see the appendix).

Among other things, this state of affairs raises questions about whether traditional health practitioners, and bonesetters in particular, are being mobilized to the extent necessary in settings with high burdens of injury. Resorting to traditional bonesetters can be framed as an increasingly relevant adjunct to clinical care in Guatemala, since rates of injury there seem to be increasing across the board. With careful planning, bonesetters might help fill certain gaps in service, as researchers have proposed in some underserved African settings (Dada et al. 2009; Owumi et al. 2013; Thanni 2000). Impeding this employment in underserved Guatemalan settings may be the health centers themselves, since these facilities enact models of care that privilege formally impartible health knowledge, something quite dissimilar from bonesetters' knowledge. The centers also exert an outsized influence over local peoples' view of the public health system. Health centers remain state signposts as much as medical signposts, and with their upgrade to twenty-four-hour *centros de atención* in 2009, they may be expanding their local reach even more. And with this change, they are also poised to loom even larger over local curers—bonesetters, midwives, and so on—individuals inhabiting the interstices of the system represented by the centers.

As more Guatemalans lose their lives and livelihoods to injuries each year, more families face catastrophic emotional and economic blows. Bonesetters have helped soften those blows in many cases. But just as injuries strike Guatemalans in myriad ways, Maya bonesetters have developed quite different ways of treating those who survive injury and want to improve their situation.

Different Tendencies, Different Chapters: A Look Ahead

There are two main Maya approaches to bonesetting, as I mentioned earlier, each with its own forms of diagnosis and treatment. I discerned these two bonesetting tendencies over the course of my research and found that while one takes an empirical approach, the other prioritizes a more sacred view of the craft. Each approach takes the client's recovery as its end goal, but each approach has developed pathways to this that are as distinct from each other as Comalapa is from the lakeside towns.

To be a bonesetter in Middle America means that one must apply direct manual treatments to people who have been injured. Approached by people beset with pain and immobility, bonesetters try singling out the physical cause of the problem and ameliorating it, if they can. This takes first and foremost a manual sensibility, so pragmatic diagnostic and treatment skills are the mainstay of these bonesetters' tool kits. With so many bonesetters relying on these skills, the empirical mode of bonesetting remains the prevailing one in the region. Less common, but still important in certain places, are bonesetting traditions that couple manual techniques with an emphasis on supernatural elements. Many bonesetters working in this sacred mode in Guatemala use objects that were revealed to them in dreams or that were bequeathed by family members. Discovery of these objects typically marks out bonesetters as legitimate practitioners, and they use the objects together with manual methods to diagnose and treat physical problems. For the most part, Maya bonesetters articulate their knowledge in one of these two registers. So deeply imprinted are these differences on Maya bonesetting that they affect how parts of this book are structured.

This introductory chapter discussed the importance of bonesetting and the need for more research about it. It then spelled out some basics about the research setting and gave a preview of the injury context in which bonesetters work. Chapter 1 walks the reader through some of the known history of bonesetting, looking at how bonesetting traditions have taken shape on a global scale since antiquity. Subsequent chapters then explore each of the two main Maya bonesetting traditions. Since part of the goal of this book is to show how each tradition is locally meaningful, chapters 2 and 3 bring the reader closer to individual bonesetters and their experiences. These two chapters will also demonstrate how bonesetters (whatever their background) know that their clients do not exist in social isolation, and how these practitioners endeavor to return their clients to their family and work roles as quickly as possible.

My intention here will be not to provide entire case histories of injury, treatment, and resolution but to provide context for the therapeutic encounters that bonesetters carry out. This includes exploring what the encounters reveal about Maya outlooks on health. Chapter 4 examines how Maya bonesetters are trying to inhabit a health workspace now populated by many formal providers and their technologies. The most pressing of these technologies, radiography, is of special interest here, because its use presupposes a superior visual way of diagnosing and reifying injury. The book's conclusion restates the importance of bonesetting amidst other healing specialties and reiterates some of the challenges confronting bonesetting in parts of the world where clinicians are deciding to either oppose the activity or somehow incorporate it into primary care. It also looks ahead to possible changes in Maya bonesetting, many of which are also traceable to its interactions with biomedicine. Bonesetting practices in different communities may fare differently over the long term, depending on whether pressures from institutional actors force changes in bonesetters' work practices and on how these changes might in turn affect public confidence in the craft. Regardless of whether individual Maya bonesetters today feel pressured to change by biomedicine, they say bonesetting has been around for many years. It is no less an ancestral inheritance than language, farming, weaving, or midwifery. That bonesetting is an old craft is certainly true on a global scale. This becomes immediately apparent once we take evidence from people of different cultures, including Mesoamerican ones, into account.

CHAPTER 1

Bonesetting over Time

To better understand how bonesetting occupies such an important place in Maya healing, it will help first to see how bonesetting has existed on a global scale for a very long time. People have always run the risk of injury and have had to deal with injury once it happens. This was as true in antiquity as it is today (Majno 1975). It should not be surprising, then, to find that different peoples left either records or other evidence showing that they tried to handle fractures, dislocations, sprains, and other injuries when the need arose (Peltier 1990). Nor should it surprise us that specialists often reached considerable heights of skill and sophistication when addressing bodies in pain and that they achieved this quite early in written history, if not earlier. We are left not with the question of whether bonesetting existed among earlier peoples but with what forms it took and in what contexts it developed. Available evidence from some of the more dominant traditions lets us track how bonesetting took shape in tandem with medicine and surgery in the cultural settings where it proved essential.

Bonesetting in Antiquity

Some of the earliest documented interest in bonesetting can be found in the traditions of Egypt. In documents such as the Edwin Smith Papyrus, for instance, fracture injuries are presented as something that a physician can treat, along with certain other diseases and infirmities of the body (Breasted 1980). Although this papyrus dates to the seventeenth century BC, the information it contains was likely in circulation much earlier, making this document a useful window into how Egyptian physicians, from an early period, made empirical assessments of injured bodies and applied their skills accordingly. Those who used this papyrus as a medical guide evidently believed that to treat problems of the body, they needed an empirical approach more than one centered on the magic and incantations so identifiable in other aspects of Egyptian life.

Widespread practices of mummification and organ removal probably added to Egyptians' empirical understandings of anatomy, and no doubt better familiarized them with the body's skeletal structure. The care they took to embalm and preserve cadavers has also let later researchers see how many Egyptians suffered from fractures and often received treatment for them (Filer 1996:86–90). Part of the story that fractures tell is that many were caused by acts of aggression. Not only do many skeletons show signs of trauma, but bone breakage in males is often on the left side of the body. Researchers have taken this to mean that the injuries were caused by right-handed assailants striking the left side of their victims' bodies and heads. Salib (1962:945), for example, noted fractures on the left radius and ulna of a male skeleton, likely created from a blow upon the left arm when it was raised defensively. "Parry fractures" such as these were among the fracture types that Egyptians treated with splints and other fixation devices. These devices appear to have been in use as early as 2730–2635 BC and were typically made from strips of wood, bark, and straw (Salib 1962: 945–946). They were usually removed before the person was buried, but could even be applied postmortem, as occurred with the Pharaoh Siptah, whose body was repaired following an intrusion into his tomb.

Egyptians, in turn, made many contributions to Greek medicine and surgery. They conveyed novel ideas, such as of the effects of food residues and putrefaction upon the body, ideas that underwent further incubation among physician-scholars of Ionia. There, especially in the polities of Knidos and Kos, medical thinking came into contact with Greek natural philosophy as it further refined the idea of humors (Saunders 1963: 22, 26–27). Greek medicine eventually took its most recognizable and enduring form in Hippocratic traditions, many of which were put to writing after the lifetime of their ostensible source, Hippocrates of Kos (ca. 460–370 BC).

While Hippocratic medicine is today best known for its theory of the four humors, it also enlarged upon existing understandings of circulation, fertility, digestion, and epidemics (see Hippocrates 1972 [1946]) and helped formalize the practice of case-centered medicine. By prioritizing an overall empirical approach to identifying infirmity, its progression, and its treatment, Hippocratic medicine set the stage for more systematic application of manual manipulation and splinting that different injuries called for. Warfare produced many injuries, but so did signature Greek activities — athletics and so forth — something that likely led to an early specialization in sports medicine. As Henry Sigerist (1971:36) reported, "There can be no doubt that accidents during sport must have been common, and that is why the surgery of fractures and dislocations was well developed in Hippocratic times [fifth and fourth centuries BC]." Greeks, like other peoples, learned about better surgical techniques as time went by and appended them to their core set of practical teachings. Consequently, their overall knowledge did not stand still during its transmission to Galen (AD 129–ca. AD 217); it continued to expand and improvise during this six-hundred-year period.

Chief among those who built upon Hippocratic teachings in the interim, especially in the arena of manual medicine, was Apollonius of Kition (ca. 60 BC). This physician trained in Alexandria, Egypt, and later worked and compiled medical knowledge in his native Cyprus, where he eventually became a court physician to King Ptolemy of Cyprus (Markatos et al. 2018). Apollonius is best remembered, though, for the treatise *Peri Arthron* (*On Joints*), a study of Hippocrates's work on articulations. The work contained excellent painted illustrations of maneuvers — many still in use today — for reducing dislocations and fractures (Markatos et al. 2018:1192).[1] This attention to classical learning as a basis for work was again seen in the hands of physician-scholars of Byzantium, who further adapted and distilled the most practical aspects of Galenic medicine (Bennett 2000). There is perhaps no better example of a worker from this period than Paul of Aegina (AD 625–690). This Saronic Islands native and student of Alexandria incorporated Hippocratic and Galenic understandings of fractures into Book Six of his *Epitome Medicae Libri Septem*, a work that brought together the medical knowledge of his day and that was quoted extensively by many physicians and writers who followed (Brorson 2009:1912; Gurunluoglu and Gurunluoglu 2003:23).

Hippocratic medicine made lasting inroads into later medicine through the efforts of Arabs, Syriacs, Jews, Persians, and others who transcribed and translated many Greek medical texts in the Middle Ages (Burnett 2009). Teachings about bonesetting formed part of many resulting works, since many of their sources' authors viewed bonesetting as belonging to a suite of skills that well-rounded physician-surgeons should possess. In the work *Questions and Answers for Physicians*, for example, which is an exam or teaching guide written between AD 1200 and 1208, Abd al-Azız Al-Sulamı devotes an entire section to bonesetting (2004). Its inclusion is revealing of how many classical authors, along with their successors, were as highly regarded for their knowledge about skeletal trauma as for their general knowledge of medicine. Aspiring physicians, therefore, had to know about the entire range of these authors' knowledge. For this reason they studied Hippocrates's works on fractures and articulations, as well as later works on bonesetting by al-Majusi (ca. AD 925–994), al-Razi (AD 860–932), and especially ibn-Sina (AD 980–1036), compiler and author of the highly influential *al-Qanun*. And as works by these physicians, scholars, and translators became more available in Europe, they opened the way for more teaching about surgery in schools of medicine there (Watt 1972:67).

From al-Khowarizmi (ca. AD 780–850), who produced a foundational mathematical treatise, came an additional development of note. The title of his chief work, *al-Kitāb al-mukhtaṣar fi ḥisāb al-jabr wal-muqābala (The Compendious Book on Calculation by Completion and Balancing)* (ca. AD 825), supplied the term *al-jabr*, the source of the word "algebra." Literally "the redintegration or reunion of broken parts" (Gandz 1926:437), algebra also came to refer to bonesetting, since it dealt with restoration and completion of things incomplete. Bonesetter-surgeons were thus known as *algebristas* in Spain from before the fifteenth century until at least the seventeenth century (Alvar Ezquerra 2005:15; Brouard Uriarte 1972:248–249; Granjel 1971:121). And even though algebristas were not formally part of the surgical establishment, seventeenth-century King Philip III ordered that all those seeking the title of surgeon should study with an algebrista for a year (Granjel 1971:122–123). This ruling, however, may not have been implemented. The work of these bonesetters' counterparts in sixteenth-century England, accordingly, was advertised as "Algebra and Bonesetting" (Green 1958:45).[2]

Building upon their predecessors' work, Galenic scholars and practitioners availed themselves of what earlier knowledge existed and took it further. They laid the foundation for university-based medicine in the West and provided the bibliographic footing that was to remain in place until at least the seventeenth century. We can see in their case how medical ideas underwent further germination within a system that was initially based on outside learning.

Successive waves of learning also characterize medical and surgical practice in Asia, particularly in India and China, where bonesetting has a long documented history. In India, where bonesetting developed primarily within an Ayurvedic framework, works on bone fracture and treatment are traceable back to an early period, perhaps 1500 BC (Bali and Ebnezar 2012:141). Classics from this period not only describe the reduction of fractures but provide information on the devices healers used, such as bandages and slings. They also prescribe posttreatment therapies to be applied in tandem with special diets (Bali and Ebnezar 2012:148). Writings from five hundred years later elaborate further on the fractures and dislocations a bonesetter should recognize and the ways they should be treated. Specialized forms of "traction, manipulation by local pressure, opposition and stabilisation, and immobilisation," applied in line with understandings about vital points in the body (Unnikrishnan et al. 2010:185), continued to undergird the doctrinally structured bonesetting traditions in the subcontinent in later centuries.

Specialists in China also advanced bonesetting practices from an early period. Their interest in these practices was at times expressed in medical treatises, the best known of which is *The Yellow Emperor's Classic of Medicine* (Maoshing 1995). This work is attributed to the Yellow Emperor Huang Di, ca. 2600 BC, though it may date to much later in time, 300–100 BC. In it we see some of the earliest Chinese references to manual manipulation and splinting, together with the extensive use of acupuncture. Significantly, the treatise underscores how a primary purpose of massage is to move energy around the body and stimulate its flow (Maoshing 1995: 107, 148), not simply to move bones and tissues. To practice bonesetting during this period, then, was to subscribe to an energy-centric system that became further institutionalized in later centuries. During the Song and Yuan Dynasties (tenth to fourteenth centuries AD), for instance, as Tui na massage became more formalized among Imperial physicians, bonesetting techniques became further refined (Pritchard 2010:84). They underwent renewed attention during the Ming Dynasty (fourteenth to seventeenth centuries AD), consolidating the bonesetter-massager's place in China's medical landscape.

As in India (Unnikrishnan 2010:185), much of the need for bonesetting skill in China grew from a high incidence of traumatic injury caused not only by warfare and accidents but also by martial arts practice. That bonesetting had been common practice among people involved in wider Asian martial arts traditions (Narangoa and Altanjula 2006:238; Pritchard 2010:5) speaks to more than just the hard realities of training, however. It is also suggestive of its modes of transmission. Together with the philosophical and physical skill set that masters taught, bonesetting and massage became part of the knowledge base passed from master to pupil in martial arts settings, allowing many interpretations of prevalent bonesetting systems to flourish at the front lines of injury.

Tibet and Mongolia, where manual manipulation practices also reach into antiquity, have likewise witnessed a mélange of factors bearing on local bonesetting. This is particularly true in Tibet. There, where early healing practices can be traced to Bon traditions, we see a later and long infusion of Indian teachings, beginning in the third century AD (Kapur 2016:147). Tibet's kings regularly invited foreign physicians, encouraging active dialogue between native, Indian, Chinese, and Galenic traditions. One outcome of this was the creation of Tibetan medicine's foundational text, the *Gyud Chi*. Compiled in the eighth century AD by a court physician, it paid ample attention to anatomy and physiology (Kapur 2016: 148). Tibetan medicine's influence (largely via Buddhism) also extended to Mongolia, where Tibetan herbal medicine and pharmacopoeia became very important (Narangoa and Altanjula 2006:237). This influence continued on to Buryatia, southern Siberia, in the eighteenth century AD (Bolsokhoyeva 2007:335, 341), where Tibetan texts were translated into Classical Mongolian and used in Buryat medical education. Although much of Mongolia's herbal medicine can be traced to Tibet, Mongolia and Tibet each had their own early bonesetting traditions. Mongolian bonesetting had early ties to shamanism, and the authority to set bones often hinged on one having ancestral ties to bonesetter-shamans (Narangoa and Altanjula 2006:237–239). In its Buryat expressions, Mongolian medicine became respected not only for bonesetting but also for practices of bloodletting, cauterization, and wound care (Bolsokhoyeva 2007:337).

Bonesetting is indebted to these many practitioners and scholars not only because they validated its importance for people but also because they encoded it into systems that, to greater or lesser degrees, formed the basis of later medical and surgical traditions that eventually became orthodoxy in their respective parts of the world. Western and Eastern medicines have continued the tradition of mapping onto existing systems. And just as bonesetting had an early established presence in the Old World, it was also prevalent in early America, especially Mesoamerica, making its signatures there worth exploring.

Therapeutic Treatment of Bones in the Mesoamerican Archaeological Record

Bonesetting has only a partially documented history in Middle America. But in the absence of written records, skeletal remains can suggest a lot about past bonesetting practices. When archaeological bones show signs of trauma and subsequent healing, it usually points to deliberate attempts to treat those injuries when the victim was still alive. Interred bones thus provide some of our earliest, albeit incomplete, glimpses of how people have long turned to each other for help. By placing the spotlight on archaeological bone remains, I hope to convey a sense of how far back bonesetting extends in Middle America.

Bonesetting is probably of great antiquity in Middle America, and skeletal remains are a prime source of information about its practice and distribution. We can also use them to extrapolate something of its cultural importance.[3] But bones reveal bonesetting only insofar as they can bear the imprint of a variety of human activities, in general. Visible patterns of bone wear, asymmetry, and robusticity, for example, have been linked to gendered occupational activities such as heavy-load lifting and food processing (Wanner et al. 2007). At the same time, well-developed muscle attachment points on bone can signal intense overall mobility (Cucina et al. 2015:154) or muscularity (Hernández and Márquez 2006:140) in certain individuals. Diseases (i.e., anemia, osteitis, osteoarthritis, and osteoporosis) also leave their imprint on bone, as can some cases of traumatic injury (Dávalos Hurtado 1970; Wright and Chew 1998). When evidence of traumatic injury on bone appears associated with postinjury manipulation and healing, we can usually infer that some injury reduction took place, or was at least attempted. That is, if bones with signs of injury are found that appear to have been handled after the injury, and if they show some intended mending, then it is reasonable to conclude that someone tried to set them. Examining bones of this type and seeing their degree of alignment and fusion, among other things, can give us a glimpse of a treatment outcome in that one case. If other examples of therapeutically handled bones are also taken into account, they might together give us a better sense of the injuries curers such as bonesetters tried to treat, when they did this, and among which groups of people.

Still, while bones can provide useful biological and cultural information (Storey 1992:161; Whittington 1989), there are limits to what we can learn from them. Wood et al. (1992) have cautioned that while paleopathological analysis of bone can provide detailed information about the skeletons of specific people who died at particular times and whose skeletons were preserved, it cannot be used to extrapolate the general state of health of the group. Skeletal specimens drawn from a given group are typically too limited in number, sex, and ages to reveal much about the group's morbidity and mortality rates, or even the life expectancy of its members (Wright and Chew 1998:934). Even the lesions visible on bones might represent only a particular stage of a disease's progression or a particular moment following recovery from traumatic injury, and do not necessarily tell us what other health conditions were present in that individual's life or what the individual died from. Furthermore, according to Mays (2018:15), the severity and range of disease in archaeological skeletons do not always accord with the severity of disease in living populations. This means that skeletal materials from the later twentieth century, which are often used to reference much older bone specimens, are not likely to show the more severe, untreated expressions of disease such as the arthropathies found in archaeological populations. It may not be possible, therefore, to reference the signs on older bones to available specimens in museums or anatomical collections, limiting our ability to interpret them.

Bones help us even less when we try to identify whether any healing rituals were applied to the persons whose skeletons we can now examine; while ritual activities might leave a visible signature on some bones (such as molded skulls and filed teeth), we cannot see the rituals themselves. In the same way, we cannot view the fused ends of broken bones and assess whether they received any ritual attention or how much of it. Neither can we directly determine whether living bones were considered sacred. Nevertheless, because people have long been therapeutically interested in bone, and because this shows on many skeletal specimens, we have something to work with when it comes to gauging the kinds of injuries people have suffered and the cultural importance they placed on treating them.

Signs of Trauma and Treatment

Bones with apparently healed fractures are found in some archaeological collections, though specimens can be few in any one collection. The paucity of bones showing disease lesions or fractures in any one collection, and the noncentralized reporting of these across collections, has made it hard to measure health problems in ancient groups (Buikstra and Cook 1980:435). Researchers also disagree about exactly which diseases left scars on particular bone specimens, and this situation further limits our ability to create health profiles of different groups (Cucina et al. 2015: 160–161). The record nonetheless shows that bones received treatment from an early period. Skeletons exhibiting trauma span the Middle American timeline, registering the presence of injury even among the region's Preclassic inhabitants. When such skeletons occur early on, they not only indicate the antiquity of trauma but also can suggest how human exposure to injury has changed over time.

Taking Tehuacan Preclassic skeletal materials into account, for example, James Anderson (1965:497) indicates that skeletons with healed fractures occur in earlier levels there more than in later levels, suggesting that "the marked decrease in evidence of trauma [at later levels] no doubt reflects the adoption of a sedentary way of life and an easier one."[4] With increasing sedentariness, the likelihood of traumatic injury presumably decreases, even though, as Jorge Luis Villacorta Cifuentes (1976:130–133) argues for early Guatemalans, living conditions remained rough after this time, causing injuries.[5] As would be expected, not all fracture treatments were fully successful, and Late Preclassic skeletal materials show this. A right tibia from Cuello, Belize, thus bears a healed fracture at its distal end, but a left femur fractured at its distal end, also from the site, shows misalignment with an overgrown callus (Robin 1989:338, 371). Five other healed fractures have been found in a Cuello mass burial, those of a foot phalanx, capitate (a bone located in the center of the wrist), lunate, distal left radius ("Colles" fracture), and left radius and ulna ("parry" fracture) (Saul and Saul 1997:43). The latter fracture, involving two bones, was misaligned. The fact that only male specimens in this site had fractures and the high incidence of healed fractures in a mass burial group suggest to Julie Mather Saul and Frank Saul (1997) that trauma linked to combat or sports was something faced by males in particular. Be that as it may, traumatic injury, and its treatment, remained a fact of life for later Middle Americans in general.

Classic period skeletons subsequently exhibit, among other signs of compromised health, healed fractures, as reported for Caracol (Chase 1994: 132) and Piedras Negras burials (Coe 1959:125). Likewise, Frank Saul's (1972:50) study of osteological material at Altar de Sacrificios specifically documents a clavicle and an ulna, bones frequently broken in the human body, showing postfracture healing. In the Guatemalan highlands, meanwhile, among T. Dale Stewart's (1949) Early to Middle Classic findings at Kaminaljuyu' is a left femur showing deformity. He suggests a possible case of greenstick fracture, albeit poorly healed. Exhibiting a better healing outcome is a humerus from the Terminal Classic site of Xochicalco in central Mexico. Stewart (1956:140) reported that the bone bore signs of a healed fracture with minimal deformity.

Later skeletons also show signs of injury and treatment. In Yucatán, for example, Fry's (1956:555) Postclassic Mayapan specimens include a fractured adult right femur with apparent healing. The distal part of the bone had moved laterally and posteriorly. Another Postclassic or Postcontact adult femur, examined in a rock-shelter near Lake Mensabak, Chiapas, also showed evidence of breakage and mending. This left femur, though, displayed a midshaft break that had healed with such excellent alignment that its examiners surmised it had been set with medical-quality stabilization and splinting (Cucina et al. 2015:156). Researchers of the early colonial frontier site Tipu, Belize, also identified trauma in Maya skeletons, but they reported that it was relatively rare in the 457 skeletons they examined and was most commonly found on tibiae (Cohen et al. 1994:126).

Other skeletons and skulls found at these and other places exhibit antemortem fractures, but their degree of healing is indeterminate. These include material from Chiapa de Corzo, Chiapas (Jaén Esquivel 1968: 74); Nebaj, Guatemala (Stewart 1951:87); Sarteneja, Belize (Kennedy 1983:359–361); Altar de Sacrificios, Guatemala (Saul 1972:51); and Chichén Itzá, Yucatán (Hooton 1973:277). While the matter of whether pre-Columbian bones show syphilis is beyond my scope of coverage, Stewart (1953) has noted the similarity between signs of syphilis and signs of normal trauma on bone. In his study of skeletons at the Guatemalan site of Zaculeu, Stewart (1953:300) conjectured that the lesions found on two tibiae and two ulnas from the Classic period may have been caused by either bone syphilis or trauma. He favored the latter possibility, however. Stewart (1956:140) also ventured that the bowed tibiae of a person with a fractured humerus, found at Xochicalco, might indicate an underlying syphilitic condition.

These osteological findings do not provide us with firm conclusions about pre-Columbian skeletal health and bonesetting, other than to say that early Middle Americans dealt with trauma. People probably valued bonesetting skill, even when fractures were not fully reduced in the end; attempted treatment was likely more important than inaction. The cultural dimensions of bonesetting among early Middle Americans remain hard to discern, though. We are left with an incomplete chronological picture of early bonesetting, even in the Maya region from which much skeletal data derives. As we enter into the colonial period, during which time Spanish observers took notice of native healing practices, the information gap closes slightly.

Colonial-Period Observations of Bonesetters

The work of Spanish chroniclers, especially that of Fray Bernardino de Sahagún (1974) in the sixteenth century, provides a useful look at different Nahua bonesetting practices. Sahagún describes how broken bones needed to be first "pressed, stretched, joined" and the limbs stabilized with cloth, splints, and cords (1974:153,161). Exposed broken bones might even be treated by the insertion of a resinous stick into the intramedullary cavity, followed by the binding of the wound (1974:153). Several of his descriptions stress the need to lance inflamed areas with an obsidian blade, as well as the need to apply urine, maguey sap, pine resin, *toloa* (*Datura* spp.), and other substances to the injuries (Sahagún 1974: 140, 153, 158, 161). The use of native plants and of technologies such as the sweat bath, together with the manual manipulation of injuries, suggested strong continuities between pre-Columbian and early colonial Mexican bonesetting practices.

A later Spanish cleric took a distinct approach when writing about Nahua bonesetters. Hernando Ruiz de Alarcón (1984 [1629]) described bonesetters in the seventeenth century, but primarily to voice his ire against them. Although he detailed how the healers he accosted would mend and splint broken bones, he was much more interested in exposing and extirpating what he considered their illegitimate ritual practices (1984:190–192). He disparaged many aspects of their work, among them the pricking of the sufferer's back with a viper's tooth and the practice of addressing the broken bone as the Mictlan-bone, or "bone of Hell," as he called it (1984:190). That as many Nahuas continued treating as many injuries as actually did, in the climate of fear that priests such as Ruiz de Alarcón perpetuated, is worthy of note.

The form pre-Columbian and colonial bonesetting took among Mayas and other non-Nahua groups, meanwhile, remains much less clear. For instance, in a brief passage in the *Pop wuj*, the K'iche' Maya account of creation, an invoked Grandfather and Grandmother mention that they set bones, even though this is not their primary activity in the narrative.[6] We later get a glimpse of colonial-period Maya bonesetters in a Kaqchikel Maya language dictionary produced in the mid-eighteenth century by Fray Thomás de Coto (Coto 1983). In his *Thesavrvs verborv*, the Franciscan Coto makes reference to a "vikol bak: el qfuej asi conçierta huesos" (*wikol bak*: he who thus arranges bones) (1983:107), and "vikol bak: el q[ue] compone o conçierta los huesos" (wikol bak: he who fixes or arranges bones) (1983: 132). He provides the latter definition of a repairer of bones as a subdefinition of a "ÇURUJANO o çirujano: Ah a3om [ajq'om]," (surgeon) (1983: 132). Coto thus conveys the understanding of bonesetting as an expression of surgery, a view prevalent at the time. Elsewhere in his dictionary he refers to the practice of applying splints, *aq*, to broken limbs. Coto describes these objects as "las tablillas en q[ue] ponen el brazo o pierna quebrada" (the little boards in which they place the broken arm or leg) (Coto 1983:528), but he does not connect their use directly to the work of vikol bak (wikol baq).

Much later in time, as part of Ralph Roys's compendium of lowland Maya medicine drawn from seventeenth- and eighteenth-century Maya texts, he (1976 [1931]:xxii) describes how the *kax-bac*, or "bone binder," uses massage and manipulation to cure "fractures, sprains, dislocations and contusions." He notes that Maya bone binders also use poultices made from leaves or roots and that a plant called "bone-remedy" has for centuries been applied to injuries. So though a few references to Maya colonial bonesetting practices do exist (Orellana 1987:106), nowhere do Maya bonesetters receive the attention that Nahua bonesetters received from colonial Spanish writers. Today's limited documentation of Maya bonesetting thus echoes the brief coverage of this topic by much earlier chroniclers and observers.

CHAPTER 2

Empirical Forms of Maya Bonesetting

Bonesetting in San Juan Comalapa

By the time the bus rumbles to a stop in San Juan Comalapa, most of its passengers are tired either from standing in the aisle or from squeezing four-deep onto seats designed for two. But with the airbrake now announcing their trip's end, the riders collect their baskets, backpacks, and children and move down the stairwell. Those passengers who were lucky enough to get a seat would have gotten a good view of the forested hills, cultivated fields, and ravines marking the approach to town. They would have seen the cypresses and pines give way to growing numbers of cinder-block houses until, having reached the center of town, the only trees left to be seen were those populating distant hilltops just outside Comalapa's urban footprint.

The passengers disembarking these days are not as dusty as they used to be when busing down this road, and for this they can thank road-improvement projects carried out in the late 1990s. Many locals claim that these changes brought more growth to the town, as shown in part through the many more stores, cars, and even motorized three-wheel taxis now buzzing through the streets than before. But even though Comalapa was never frozen in time, locals lament that the rapid change of pace means that their children will never know the sleepier town they themselves grew up in. Youngsters today are probably more likely to find a future in Guatemala City than they are to live and raise a family here like their parents did. Their outlooks on the world are no doubt also affected by the increasing media connectivity and computer usage that feature in their lives. One thing that has not changed with the visual and digital transformation of Comalapa, though, is how Comalapans continue relying on bonesetters and other informal caregivers.

Despite the emergence of new patterns of work and living in Comalapa, the need for bonesetters shows no signs of abating. This is because the way bodies move through more spaces than before, be they footpaths or highways, has actually meant that bodies continue to need at least as much manual care as before, care that the town's bonesetters are there to provide. This chapter provides a look at a Kaqchikel Maya bonesetting tradition built on the idea that physical problems require physical solutions. Its practitioners live like everyone else around them, with nothing to distinguish them as having any clinical training or special insights into the supernatural. And because they live like those around them, they are all too aware of how swiftly injury and debility can strike and how it can afflict entire households. Bonesetters deal with the problems of their neighbors because their neighbors trust them to deliver tangible, physical results. As a community home to an empirical form of bonesetting, San Juan Comalapa pays witness to how pragmatic considerations take center stage when bonesetters diagnose and treat clients. One can see that bonesetters spend a lot of time palpating and massaging during treatments and very little time, if any, praying. Theirs is a work that grows both from experience and from personal familiarity with pain, making their craft far more individualized than the work of clinicians could be.

We see something of each bonesetter's signature in the approaches and techniques that individual bonesetters favor. Some might be best known for manipulating limbs, others for reducing fractures. Some might use herbal mixtures, while others recommend steam treatments. Their broad range of techniques speaks to their willingness to experiment and to their desire to improve those techniques they value the most. For example, beginning in 1992 when I first met Paulino, Alejandro, and Bartolomé, I started noticing the important place massage and manipulation occupy in bonesetting. Later, when I met Eduardo and, briefly, Tonia, in 1995 I began developing a better grasp of how some workers put plants and technology to creative use. Then, when I met Rómulo and Tomás in 2000 and Lupito in 2001, they showed me the importance of decisive, often painful, body work. I watched the Comalapa bonesetters as they performed about twelve treatments. In addition to these, I received a treatment from a bonesetter. Bonesetters also told me about some forty-eight cases they had dealt with, giving me a broad sense of the physical problems they handle. Together with what many other Comalapans shared about treatments they had received or seen, the bonesetters' narratives left little doubt that a pragmatic outlook counts for a lot in their work.

Comalapa and the Empirical Approach

For the most part, Maya bonesetting is empirically driven, and what little formal training Comalapa's Kaqchikel Maya bonesetters have is equally empirical and secular. For instance, Bartolomé received some traumatological training while serving in the Guatemalan Army in the 1930s. Eduardo remembers learning some bonesetting techniques from an established curer in a neighboring Kaqchikel town, Iximche'. The remaining Comalapan bonesetters learned the work directly, as people brought difficult cases to them and they had to deal with them. Each bonesetter, though, attributes what he knows about bonesetting more to his many years of curing experience than to any one episode of treating someone. Urgent circumstance combines with limited institutional training and pragmatic skill-building into a formative experience widely seen among bonesetters in the region.

This process aligns with how the religious aspect of curing is deemphasized among bonesetters in general. On the whole, Middle American bonesetters foreground physiological etiology (Holland 1962:237–244; Orellana 1987:106). Nahuat bonesetters of Hueyapan, Puebla, for instance, reportedly "reject the idea that the supernatural world plays a role in the kinds of injuries in which they specialize" (Huber and Anderson 1996:30). For his part, the K'iche' Maya bonesetter in Chuchexic, Guatemala, "does not possess any special divine power," according to Sheila Cosminsky (1972:182). This is not to say that bonesetters do not recognize a divine component in their work. Many do acknowledge such a component, but this recognition is more pronounced in some communities than in others (Douglas 1969; Fabrega and Silver 1973; Paul 1976). For example, Comalapa Maya bonesetters similarly focus on physiological etiology, but they also remain conversant in how spiritually derived illness works. As members of the community, they understand the causes and perils of spiritual illness. But again, while most bonesetters in Comalapa recognize supernatural agency in illness and might even use some form of prayer in their work, local people do not think of them as spiritual specialists.[1]

By most accounts, bonesetters begin their craft under empirical conditions, and they later practice it empirically. Many bonesetters in Comalapa, San Pedro La Laguna, and San Juan La Laguna describe how they were initially summoned to help an injured person, sometimes when out in the fields or far from home. Some even had to treat their own injuries. They then developed their treatment abilities by attending to more people who came looking for them in their homes. In about half of Middle American indigenous groups, moreover, bonesetter novices also learn from more experienced bonesetters, possibly family members (Paul and McMahon 2001:247). An intense physicality thus characterizes the bonesetters' work from their first, formative moments onward. So pragmatic and non-ritualized is the work of most bonesetters that in Guatemala, where there are many formal religious divisions, bonesetters who happen to be of a particular Christian denomination often get sought by clients of other denominations. Their work allows them to keep a secular reputation in the midst of local religious fractiousness, a point I will return to in chapter 3.

Other features of this craft also recall its empirical basis, including the ways bonesetters provide physical treatment during moments of public need and how they use pragmatic resources. Following Guatemala's devastating 1976 earthquake, for example, Maya bonesetters received more injured people than ever. The bonesetters Alejandro, Bartolomé, and Tomás recall the many injuries they had to treat, the many broken bodies people brought them. They had to deal with many injuries in a short time, something they had not done before but that taught them a lot. By treating people of different ages, for instance, they got a good sense of how bodies heal at different rates. This experience dovetailed with what they saw later in their careers, when they had to treat injured soccer players and other young people whose bodies healed more quickly than those of older people.

As another indication of their empirical approach, most Comalapans who perform manual body work also perform a lot of abdominal or body massage. When they do this work, moreover, they are usually guided by non-Western views of the body. For example, many Comalapans say that the stomach contains a pouch that is home to very active naturally occurring worms. In the case of severe stomach pain, then, the massagers must move the wayward worms back into their pouch to ease the upset stomach. This vermicular symbiosis has been noted elsewhere in Guatemala (Acevedo Ligorria 1986:20; Rosenthal 1987:93) and remains the cornerstone of Comalapan abdominal illness etiology. Local bonesetters adhere to this view and may be called on to treat vermicular illness.

Bonesetters have long used both traditional and nontraditional pragmatic resources in their work. Like other curers, they recommend the home *tuj* (sweat bath) for therapeutic use. Comalapans Alejandro and Rómulo appreciate how the tuj warms the body and counteracts injurious cold *aires* that tend to target the body's joints and articulations. I will discuss aires later in this chapter. Bonesetters in the three studied towns, though, also recommend and use various commercial products.[2]

Virtually all bonesetters, for example, use the store-bought preparations Pomada GMS, Balsámico GMS, and Cofal at some point, products that are rubbed onto the skin and can help lubricate the body for manipulation. They also recommend the pain-relieving *pomada* (pomade) Nodol to clients who need an analgesic. Most bonesetters also make use of drugs that are taken internally and that are known by their brand names.[3] Tomás sometimes suggests that clients with fractures buy Indocin and Anatran because they act "like a vitamin, [for] the bone, so that the bone will fuse." Paulino, meanwhile, recommends Mejoral because it counteracts the "cold" in the body caused by pain, showcasing a "hot" property that Alejandro also attributes to the salve Balsámico GMS. For relief of pain and inflammation, bonesetters in San Pedro La Laguna and San Juan La Laguna make use of Dolofin, Dolorin, Dolo-Fenil, and Neo-Melubrina. In Comalapa other drugs that also ease inflammation and rheumatic symptoms, such as Indocin and Reumetan, are likewise used or recommended by bonesetters.[4] A bonesetter in San Pedro La Laguna also reportedly uses Reumetan. One San Pedro bonesetter whom I will introduce in chapter 3 even administers an injectable form of the NSAID (nonsteroidal anti-inflammatory drug) Dolo-Fenil to some clients (Hinojosa 2004c:119). Clients are administered these products in the course of receiving the bonesetter's manual treatment.

During my early interactions with Comalapa bonesetters, I learned about another nontraditional resource, an unexpected one, entering the bonesetters' space: some clients bring X-ray images of their injuries. I later found this to be true for bonesetters of the lakeside towns as well. But while most Maya bonesetters consider X-ray images interesting, they do not consider them necessary for their work. In fact, radiographs have become most useful in recent years in confirming for the client the bodily condition that the bonesetter first detects with his hands. So sure are bonesetters of their manual diagnostic method that in some cases, they might even encourage a client who doubts the bonesetter's manual diagnosis to take X-rays of his injuries (Hinojosa 2004b). As I discuss in chapter 4, this imaging is meant to confirm the bonesetter's findings, not replace his methods.

Injuries and the Treatment Encounter

The Maya world of work can and does produce many injuries among men and women. The bonesetters I learned from report that most people approach them with *golpes*, a term referring to injuries ranging from deep tissue bruises to joint sprains. Other people present to them with more serious joint problems involving stiffness, swelling, and extreme pain, often due to dislocations. Fracture cases are sometimes brought to Comalapan bonesetters, though not all bonesetters will attempt to reduce them. In each case, it is up to the bonesetter to determine the nature of the injury and whether he thinks he can help the injured.

This assessment usually takes place in the bonesetter's home. If the person seeking help has relatively minor injuries or discomforts, he or she might first greet the bonesetter, speak informally with him, and only later turn the conversation to the problem. If the person seeking help arrives with a serious problem such as a fracture or a dislocation or is in great pain, the injury will be addressed immediately. Bonesetters listen carefully to the client's account of how the injury occurred, then visually check the injury site for edema, color, and protrusions. If the bonesetter can move the limb, he or she will try to determine its range of motion.

Bartolomé, Rómulo, Tomás, and other bonesetters who do treat fracture cases then perform the difficult and painful task of realigning the bones. The individuals that brought the injured person to the bonesetter are expected to help. They might simply steady the person while the bonesetter works, or they might have to hold him or her firmly from behind if the bonesetter has to pull on an arm or leg. Then, depending on the type of fracture, the bonesetter may simply wrap the area with a gauze or cloth, or he or she may immobilize the limb using materials such as cardboard or sticks, something usually indicated for fractured long bones. One Comalapan bonesetter whom Icú Perén included in his study (1990) would even apply hard casts, but most bonesetters prefer immobilizing arrangements that can be removed easily, which enables checking the injury site a few days after the initial reduction to examine its alignment and progress. Bonesetters will massage the area to determine the bones' position and to correct it, if necessary. They may have to do this several times, depending on the type of break and on how well the client has been keeping it immobilized since it was first treated.

Dislocations must also be properly reduced by the bonesetters, and this can also be painful. But while these injuries may not be life threatening, they are still considered serious. First, they are clearly painful and debilitating, and this alone makes them dangerous for a family's economic future: if the breadwinners cannot move in order to work, everyone in the household will suffer. Second, dislocations can worsen and become harder to correct because of the way the body is said to react to them. The bone-setters Alejandro and Paulino say that when there is a dislocation, a "meat" begins growing inside the joint, making treatment difficult. This happened to Paulino's granddaughter, who tripped in a hole while playing at school and dislocated her knee. Her manual treatment got delayed, and she even-tually required surgery in Guatemala City to remove the growth from her knee and to repair the damage.

But whether diagnosing a client's injury for the first time or offering follow-up care for fractures or dislocations, the Maya bonesetter relies on his hands. Of primary importance is what the injured body can directly communicate to the bonesetter. To make this communication possible, the bonesetter's hands must perform a special operation.

A Bodily Mode of Engagement

The Maya bonesetter's hands serve as his primary vehicle for diagnosis and treatment, but in a nonmechanistic way. Bonesetters stress that their hands "know" the body and can directly determine what is wrong with it, though the source of this intuition is never made clear. As Bartolomé states, "The hand knows well the injuries and the healthy bones." When a bonesetter places his hands on a body, therefore, his hands guide him, and not the other way around.

Bonesetters cannot usually explain how their hands achieve this way of knowing, but they insist it is untaught. The hands slowly actualize this as they make contact with suffering bodies. Elsewhere in the Maya area, the hands' ability to diagnose and heal limbs is sometimes attributed to the aid of spirit helpers (Paul 1976:78), but this is not the case in Comalapa. One researcher did say, however, of Comalapa Maya bonesetters, "They all commented that they feel more secure when they invoke God in prayer, and that an inexplicable force takes control of them and guides their hands and mind" (Icú Perén 1990:53). This proclivity is reflected in how Rómulo links his hands' abilities to his mind and to God. Talking about his hands he says, "Those are the tools that God has gifted me. The hands, that is the best tool I have, and the mind, because you have to focus with the mind, the hands, and the power of the Lord. He is these three things. First the Lord, second the hands, and third is intelligence." He here stresses the larger set of forces within which his hands work and that God enables, but he later adds that the most important confluence of agency centers on "la mano en contacto con la mente" (the hand in communication with the mind). For him, the hands' link to the (nonconscious) mind is of more immediate practical importance than their link to any other reality, super-natural or otherwise.

This hand-based way of knowing contrasts with the path to curing legitimacy marking other healing specialties in Comalapa. Midwives and soul specialists usually report that something awakened them to their healing work, or confirmed for them their need to do it (Hinojosa 2015). This impetus may have been a series of dreams, an unexpected event, or a set of strange occurrences. With one exception (that of Tomás), the local bonesetters I met do not report having experienced any portents. They generally begin their work by urgent circumstance, out of immediate ne-cessity (e.g., the 1976 earthquake), and without apparent divine election. While some bonesetters in Comalapa may have experienced events they felt confirmed them in their work, they seldom attribute a spiritual quality to them in the way that other healers do.[5] Bonesetters instead admit that circumstance plays the greatest role in launching their work, even if they later come to feel a singular affinity with bonesetting, placing a premium on their body telling them what they need to know about their work.

Close inspection of the bonesetting craft indeed reveals how the body can constitute a source and starting point of knowledge for bonesetters. The way a Maya bonesetter's hands directly engage the suffering body en-tails a somatic, or bodily, mode of attention that Thomas Csordas (1990, 1993, 1994) has said occurs on an unconscious level. Drawing from Maurice Merleau-Ponty (1962) and Pierre Bourdieu (1977), Csordas argues that be-fore a subject consciously objectifies the world, he or she is present in and engages it. This presence and engagement, what Csordas (1990:9), after Merleau-Ponty (1962), qualifies as "preobjective," may take place in ways not consciously perceived by the subject. Perception initially takes place not objectively and analytically but multisensorially through the body, in a way lacking the language and categories of human experience. By this process, according to Csordas (1994:6), the body comprises the existen-tial ground of culture and self, through which are laid the conditions for consciousness. In the context of this preobjective grounding, then, bodies attend to other bodies prior to their conscious elaboration as such. The body thus becomes the starting point of perception (Csordas 1993:135) and a source of knowledge of direct importance to Maya bonesetters.

This idea of embodied attention partly explains how Maya bonesetters can access critical information from their clients' bodies. When Maya bonesetters place their hands on a suffering body, information about the client's body becomes somatically available to them. Bonesetters can then achieve a direct link with that client's body. This direct engagement makes it possible for the bonesetter's hands, in a self-guided mode, to diagnose and redress the problems in the client's body. In practice, when bonesetters place their hands on clients' bodies, they often claim that their hands begin moving of their own accord, responding to the clients' bodies in ways the bonesetters do not control.[6] Maya bonesetters sometimes even liken their fingers to discrete points of consciousness, able to directly detect problems like the best X-ray machine can, as Rómulo puts it. For him, as for other bonesetters, the hands attend directly to suffering bodies without the conscious effort of the healer.

The centrality of embodied knowledge in the Maya bonesetter's work distinguishes it from biomedical practice. Whereas bonesetters rely on their hands to diagnose and treat, physicians prioritize using sophisticated tools such as X-ray machines to diagnose and, ultimately, treat injuries. Physicians criticize how Maya bonesetters have no formal training yet claim to diagnose and treat injured people. But they are even more critical of how bonesetters practice using only their hands. Local physicians find such a method to lack any scientific basis and strongly disapprove of this method to address fractures. This criticism has reconfirmed the bonesetters' belief that physicians, who bonesetters say are unable to reduce fractures, are not working in the community's best interest. For bonesetters it becomes yet another reminder of how differently Mayas and clinicians view the role of the body in healing.

Like Comalapa's bonesetters, healing and ritual specialists in other Maya communities also attend with their bodies when serving their clients, and they also report having different kinds of bodily sensations. Among K'iche' Maya, for instance, Cosminsky (1972), C. James MacKenzie (2016), and Barbara Tedlock (1992) have said that *ajq'ijab'* (calendar specialists) notice tics and other movements in their bodies when divining and attribute these to spiritual agency. The Q'anjob'al Maya diviner (La Farge 1947) and his Chorti' Maya counterpart (Wisdom 1940:344) reportedly experienced similar physical manifestations, the Chorti' diviner initiating them by applying tobacco-infused saliva to his right leg and then waiting for twitches. But while these specialists attend carefully to signs in their own bodies, signs of sometimes diffuse origin, it is different for the Kaqchikel Maya bonesetter. The bonesetter in Comalapa senses his body engaging directly with information coming specifically from the client's body. The bonesetter's body somatically "listens" to what the client's body tells it. As the bonesetter places his hands on the client's body, the healer's body apprehends the inner contours and injuries of the sufferer, and comes to coexperience the pains in the sufferer's body.

Pain and Empathy

The bodily empathy established between bonesetter and client has much in common with the deep physical bond Maya midwives are said to establish with their maternity clients. Brigitte Jordan (1993:119) takes this point further and argues that female midwives are effective at empathizing with women in the throes of labor because they are themselves women and, most often, mothers. The midwife attends to the pregnant woman's body with her own body and thus coexperiences the laboring woman's condition. This experiential feature of Maya midwifery finds resonance in the bonesetter's experience.

In some ways, like midwives, Maya bonesetters must coexperience the conditions of their clients in order to treat them. It initially surprised me that some of the Comalapan bonesetters suffered from poor health. Five of the eight bonesetters, in fact, reported having severe health problems, even disabilities. It turns out that many bonesetters have themselves been victims of musculoskeletal injuries; they have been injured and have partially recovered. They know the pain and immobility that can follow severe injuries and can empathize closely with their clients. Alejandro, for instance, suffered injuries in a 1988 car accident that left him in traction for three months. During the time I spent with him, he suffered constantly from stiffness and infections and was a recovering alcoholic. Paulino suffered in later life with severe leg immobility, edema, and incontinence. He died, probably from complications of the edema. Bartolomé, one of the most experienced of Comalapa's bonesetters, suffered continual stomach pains he attributed to a "tumor," as well as cold, cramping leg pains in the last years of his life. The bonesetter Eduardo, meanwhile, suffered injuries first to his right leg then to his left, was treated by a bonesetter, and lived for several years before succumbing to liver failure.

The bonesetters of Comalapa are no strangers to pain and injury. Among these men, it even appears as though the inability to heal oneself is requisite to an ability to heal others, in a way reminiscent of the initiatory "wounding" noted among shamanic healers (Halifax 1982). Unlike shamanic healers, though, bonesetters do not undergo the ritual death and rebirth said to mark shamanic training (Eliade 1964). But the bonesetters' bodies do suffer, and their pain is noticeable. It is striking to watch Alejandro make great efforts to walk to and from the countryside, or even to watch Bartolomé move slowly across his patio. These bonesetters can certainly empathize with people living with injuries as they move about with their own pains. Witnessing this, one might reason that having an injury or disease correlates with having healing ability or that health problems might even give rise to healing ability.[7] But since it is also the case that many nonhealers have serious health problems, another understanding of the relationship between health problems and healing ability is needed.

I suggest that instead of thinking of health problems as the mark of the healer, we should consider them as furthering the healer's ability to attend somatically to others. In persons with a heightened bodily grounding, through pain, for instance, a heightened bodily attention can emerge as a consequence. Injury, especially, may enable the bonesetter's body to better respond to and coexperience the suffering of other bodies, while at the same time legitimating for locals the bonesetter's authority to utilize his body for healing. The health problems bonesetters experience authenticate their bodies as sources of knowledge and comprise a vector through which healing knowledge is revealed.

This revealing is evident when bodily pain indicates to the bonesetter that he is acquiring healing knowledge. Thus it was for Eduardo, who felt a lot of pain in his arms when he first started working with people. As the pain gradually diminished, he felt that he was progressing in his work in some way. For healers to undergo initiatory trauma is not unusual in the Maya area, but with Comalapa's bonesetters, the messages expressed through the body are usually conferred a nonspiritual quality. Their bodies manifest an intuition and knowing that are not bound up in an expressly spiritual role, even if their degree of commitment parallels what we often associate with a spiritually endorsed vocation. To the extent that some Comalapa bonesetters might see their work as a vocation, it might help to think of "vocation" not only as something resting upon a spiritual sanction per se but as an activity endorsed by a physical empathy with at least partial supernatural overtones. Bonesetting can thus be seen as a vocation, though not necessarily a spiritual one. In this framework of experience we might understand how some bonesetters partly attribute their work to a divine source. But as the following vignettes show, personal experience and creativity count for far more when it comes to their actual craft.

Bonesetters at Work

Bartolomé

Over his fifty-plus years of bonesetting, Bartolomé received many persons with painful conditions. One reason so many people came to him is he was already very well known in the community. For years he participated in the local *cofradía* (religious brotherhood) and even carried out the post of *cofrade mayor*, the chief position. This put him at the center of the signature traditionalist institution in Comalapa during the decades when traditionalist life held sway. But before he reached this distinguished public stature, he lived part of his life as a young man outside of Comalapa and as part of another institution that left an equally deep impression on him.

In 1932, at the age of seventeen, Bartolomé entered the army and was posted to the Cuartel Puerto San José on the Pacific Coast. The move took him a world away from his highland home, and it was not easy. But in his new surroundings, he discovered some new abilities. He recounted that one day a soldier twisted his ankles during training and suffered severe injury. As Bartolomé put it, the man "bent" his feet. Without providing any details, Bartolomé said that he took action and fixed the man's feet. According to Bartolomé, when the base physicians saw his work they were impressed. He even recalled a particular general telling him to go and attend to the other soldiers, and with this endorsement, he went to work in the military hospital. For the next three months, the hospital physicians taught the young conscript about various injuries, and Bartolomé was a quick study. In the end, the base planted the seed for a lifelong awakening to his work. Perhaps because he identified so much with what the army physicians taught him, he came to think of these new skills as augmenting his own natural abilities. At any rate, his practical learning sped up when he returned to his hometown.

As was true for other bonesetters, when Bartolomé was asked to diagnose and treat someone's injury, he relied on his hands. He would first apply rubbing alcohol to the person's skin and then palpate the injured area, sensing any swellings, bumps, or protrusions caused by the trauma. This, together with the client's description of what happened, would help him piece together how serious the injury was and how he needed to redress it. For most blows and dislocations, it was usually enough to massage the area with a pomada, for instance, Balsámico GMS, and then wrap it in long strips of cloth. Depending on the injury, he might then tell the person to come back in a week or so to do a follow-up massage.

When these injuries were more severe and accompanied by stiffness,

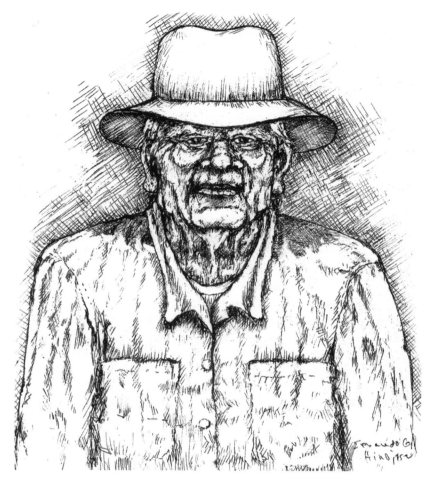

Figure 2.1. The bonesetter Bartolomé, of San Juan Comalapa. Drawing courtesy of Servando G. Hinojosa.

his method was different. He often had to apply heat during the manipulation and then tie *palitos* (stick splints) onto the limb. To illustrate how he used splints, Bartolomé described how a man with an arm injury was once brought to him. The man's arm was dislocated at the elbow and remained flexed, so the first thing Bartolomé did was heat the man's arm with water and hot, wet pads. He then massaged the arm, reduced the dislocation at the elbow, and straightened out the arm. Wrapping the arm in cotton and gauze pads, he then bound it with stick splints to keep it straight while it healed. For him, hot water made all the difference when trying to undo limb stiffness, and he argued that it also worked on fingers. Injury to the hand can make the blood "contract." "Se encoje" (it contracts or shrinks), he explained, and this causes the hand to involuntarily clench the fingers. Holding his fist in the air, he described how he used hot water and a hot massage to straighten out a client's individual fingers and how he then placed small stick splints on each of the man's fingers.

Since Bartolomé would need to revisit these injury sites, it made sense for him to use splints when treating them. But he had to be especially creative with splints in dealing with yet another case. He told me about a man he treated for a "broken back." The man had been working in the countryside when a load of wood or other heavy object fell on him. A physician in Chimaltenango examined him and said he could not help him and that he was going to die. Upon hearing this prognosis, the man's desperate family brought him to Bartolomé, who then examined him. The bonesetter found the man in a dreadful state. When he would lean forward, Bartolomé said, a bone would protrude through his back, and when he would lean back, a bone would protrude through his belly. Bartolomé had to do something.

Bartolomé first wrapped the man's entire torso, front and back, in a long gauzy sheet, and then put thick cotton padding around this. He then placed a flat board along the man's back, extending from his buttocks to his neck. To further stabilize the back, he put two narrow sheets of plywood between the man's arms and his torso, reaching from armpits to hips. He next bound the three boards together with a belt, affixing it to the man's body. Bartolomé told the man he would have to wear the entire device for a year. In the weeks that followed, the man returned to the physician in Chimaltenango. The physician asked about the splint, saying, "Who put that on you—what doctor was it?" The man told the physician that an ordinary person put it on him. According to Bartolomé's client, the physician then said that the splint should stay on. As it turned out, the injured man recovered after only three months and removed the boards much earlier than expected.

While Bartolomé's account left a lot of open questions, an important narrative thread connected this account with others he told me. Many of his clients came to him in dire straits, facing a future in which they could not move, much less work. If they had gone to clinicians who could not appreciate this prospect, it compounded their desperation. Left feeling that biomedicine had given up on them, they then turned to the bonesetter. Listening to them, placing his hands on them, and working with them, Bartolomé provided a caring option when others offered little hope. Even on his busiest days, when five people or more might come by, his knowing hands attended patiently to each body. He died at age eighty-two.

Tomás

Although decades younger than Bartolomé, the fifty-one-year-old bone-setter Tomás also draws from a deep well of knowledge. His journey began when he was fourteen or fifteen and he had to help his brother, who had injured his hand. Tomás said that after he fixed his brother's "dislocated" hand, other people noticed his skill and began talking about him. He then started working in earnest and gradually took a real liking to helping others, "so that they wouldn't have to go to the hospital." Over time, as people came to him with injuries, he expanded his skill set and learned

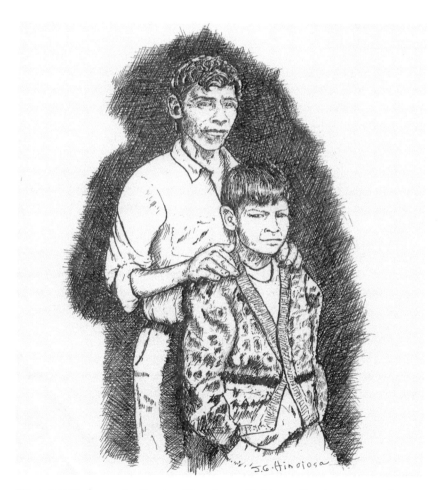

Figure 2.2. The bonesetter Tomás, of Comalapa, with his son. Drawing courtesy of Servando G. Hinojosa.

to treat fractures as well as dislocations. Today devoting himself mostly to construction work, he has seen more than his fair share of injuries in Comalapa.

When clients arrive at his door, the first thing he does is determine whether they have a break or a dislocation, and for this he turns to his hands. They deploy a knowing that comes from something greater than him. "The fingers, when I touch, I know that it's like a *don* [divine gift] . . . from God; it isn't something I've studied, nor is it a science, you know. It's something God has given me, I have a sensitive touch, when I hold with the hand, I can already find where the broken bone is; with my sensitive touch, with my sight, I can just look [and I can tell whether] it's dislocated or it's broken." His hands can find where long bones have fractured or where a bone chip has separated from the underlying bone, noting how it teeter-totters at that point. But since he also reiterates that "without touching, just by sight, just like that I can say if it's dislocated or broken," he alludes to how sight plays a role in his initial diagnostic process. The attuning of his visually driven diagnostic perception marks another way in which his skills have progressed over the years. Tomás talks about how he picks up visual cues from injury sites, but in doing so he relates that his hands sense something else: elevated temperature. He says, "The tips of my fingers already know if it's a fracture or it it's a sprain. If it's a sprain, it feels like the bone's out of place. Insofar as the bone is broken, the temperature, the color of the skin . . . it changes color, it really sparkles, it gets hot."[8]

This remark indicates that Tomás's hands attend to localized body temperature when he is trying to feel out a person's injury. In this way, he goes beyond the conventional tactile and visual assessment of deformity and edema, which entails noticing color changes and what he calls a sparkling quality in the area. Moreover, Tomás adds, when the bone is fractured he can even hear the bone ends rubbing together, making a "cluck, cluck" sound (crepitus). This description (1) suggests diagnostic parity between sight and touch and (2) proposes that while diagnosis is not quite a whole-body event, it does involve at least three senses (touch, sight, hearing), with primacy given to touch. In line with this, Guy Attewell (2016:13) expands the "sonic" dimension of embodied knowledge among bonesetters in India to include the "vocal interjections of pain" made by their clients during treatment.

Tomás attributes his overall skills to a God-given gift of touch, and he underlines this further when he says, "God has given me this don; therefore in God's name I do this work, and those people who have faith get cured." But while this comment might imply that his work is entirely divine in origin, he did not always believe he had a don. It was, in fact, only after Tomás started setting bones that he gradually came to see his abilities as a don and only at a friend's suggestion. Around 1972–1973, he spoke with a catechist about his bonesetting work, and, as he puts it, "este amigo me orientó" (this friend clarified things for me). The catechist told Tomás that maybe Tomás had a vocation and that it was a don from God. Many other local people also told Tomás this. The general message for him was "this was a gift from God, and not just any old thing." Although Tomás discovered a natural facility with bonesetting well before other people urged him to think of it as a don, appreciating its bestowal as a don provided ongoing validation for him, something needed for the work he does.

For him to treat peoples' fractures, he must have their full confidence, and over the years he has learned enough about bodies to know what different breaks are like and how long they take to heal. He describes how most arm fractures take from six to seven weeks to mend, even when the bones are totally *astillados*, splintered. If it is a smaller break, such as a *fisura* (similar to a greenstick fracture) or a *rajadita* (a smaller fracture or chip), it might take only three weeks of treatment. These fractures require him to use splints. Tomás stabilizes the injuries with small sticks or pieces of cardboard and then wraps them, noting that the areas will then quickly warm up and *se pone tieso* (become firm). After setting and splinting the injuries, he checks them every six or eight days. To do so he removes the splint, then visually and manually checks the bones' alignment and, if necessary, physically moves the bones again. He says he needs to make only four follow-up visits to the person with a fracture or dislocation, though the actual number of visits usually depends on things such as his availability on market days, intercity bus schedules, whether a client feels he is getting better, and so on.

During a follow-up house call, he shows me how he reviews a fracture repair-in-progress. The client is an approximately twenty-six-year-old woman who slipped outside her house and broke her right tibia about a week ago. She is the wife of a *moro vaquero* dancer (a member of Comalapa's traditionalist Maya dance group) I know from a few years back. Tomás sits and faces the woman as she sits on the edge of a bed. He removes a scarf that is wrapped around her lower leg; underneath it is a long strip bandage wrapped around the shin and foot, which he also removes beginning at the foot. Having removed this bandage, he begins removing another one that is fastened with clips. When this second bandage comes off, a group of oblong pieces of cardboard comes into view. These five strips of cardboard

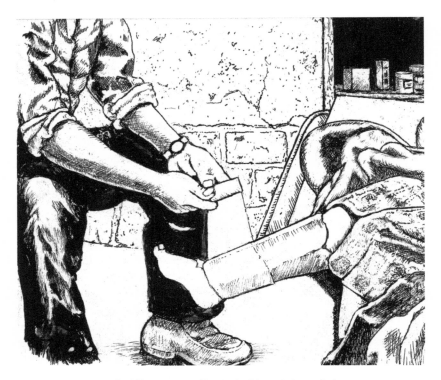

Figure 2.3. As part of a follow-up visit, Tomás, in this artistic rendering, removes wrappings he earlier applied to a woman's broken lower leg. Drawing courtesy of Servando G. Hinojosa.

run the length of her entire lower leg and are placed all around it. Two of the five strips extend down to cover the inner and outer sides of her right ankle. He then removes the strips of cardboard, showing yet another leg wrapping beneath them. The lower leg is wrapped in a long strip of towel or cloth that seems as if it was once wet but has since dried and stiffened. Once he removes the cloth, he can see the injury site.

A member of the client's family brings a bucket of water, which Tomás places beneath her leg. Using his hands, he begins wetting the lower leg, especially the ankle and foot. As he does this he says that the water is "boiled with salt . . . [I]t is for where the impact struck." He pauses to gently squeeze the ankle, then the foot, then he continues to moisten and rub the top of the foot. Tomás again moistens and rubs the lower shin, feeling out the injury, and then removes the bucket of water. After drying her leg with a fresh towel, he applies a layer of the Nodol analgesic pomada to the leg and foot, making sure to rub areas corresponding to both the tibia and fibula. Having moved his hands over the newly lubricated skin, Tomás touches the spot about two inches above the distal epiphysis, where the woman fractured her right tibia, and says, "There it is, here is the very spot where it's broken, you can feel it." With his fingers on the site he adds, "I'm telling you, the fingers are searching, they're searching for where it's damaged and I've found it right over here. Here it is, you know, the place where it's broken."

After rubbing the area a bit more, he moves his hands down to the client's foot and pivots it upward slightly. Tomás then wipes the leg, ankle, and foot with the innermost wrapping he removed earlier and readies the area for his next treatment. He reaches into his bag, bringing out a small dark jar, and then he applies a dark ointment from this jar onto the injury site. "Now we're not going to use alcohol. It's time for something else, another remedy that's more specialized for the bone that's damaged." When I ask him to tell me a little bit more about this substance, he says, "This is a, it's a remedy, it's a remedy that's . . . called a formulated mixture [*masa*

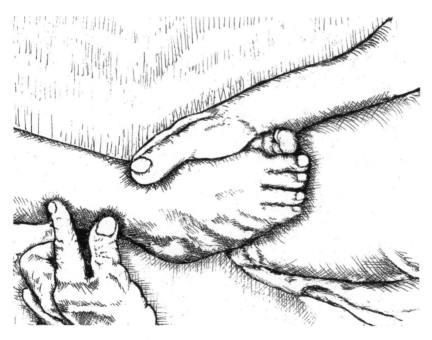

Figure 2.4. Tomás points to the fracture site just above the client's ankle. Drawing courtesy of Servando G. Hinojosa.

compuesto], it comes from a natural products specialist [naturista], yes. In here, in here they've combined seven different kinds of plants. Yes, the formulated mixture, it comes from the specialist, and it isn't found in the pharmacy; it's not in the pharmacy." He applies the tarry mixture in a wide band all around the ankle and upper part of the foot, commenting that the remedy is "hot, hot . . . it's that the bone needs heat so that it heals quickly; it will heal quickly." Satisfied that the fracture is still aligned and that he has applied enough of the hot mixture, he wipes his hands and puts away the dark jar.

Tomás next wraps the leg and foot in a new clean strip of cloth. On top of this, he places the cardboard pieces serving as a splint. This time he places a double layer of cardboard on the spot where he pointed out the tibia fracture, confirming that it's "all cardboard, yes; it's so that it will support the bone; it will cover it over." A family member steps in to support the woman's leg as he places the next layer of wrapping around the cardboard pieces, holding them in place. Once this bandaging is done, Tomás applies another layer of bandaging, covering the shin, ankle, and foot. As he does this, he chats with the client and says that taking vitamins would be a good idea. Applying clips to the bandage, he then takes the long scarf that had earlier formed the outermost wrapping and rewraps it around the leg, ankle, and foot, finally affixing it with clips. "That's it," he says, and begins collecting his things. He tells the woman and her husband that she might want to take Anatran. She nods and says she knows about the drug Indocin. He will have to come back in eight days, he says, to apply his hands again.

People sometimes go to another bonesetter before coming to him, he later tells me, or they might even go to two or three others before him. But this woman came to him first, and for him this means she will probably recover in due course. Before long, she might even be able to walk assisted to his house on a Saturday or Sunday, when he is home all day receiving people. On any given day, though, someone might come knocking frantically on his door, and even if the hour is late he will put down whatever he is doing to lend a hand.

Alejandro

Comalapans first learned that Alejandro had some healing ability when he was sixteen. As he later recounted, his grandfather had fallen and sprained his toes, and Alejandro treated him. Soon neighbors began arriving to see Alejandro, hoping he could help them with their injuries. He did what he

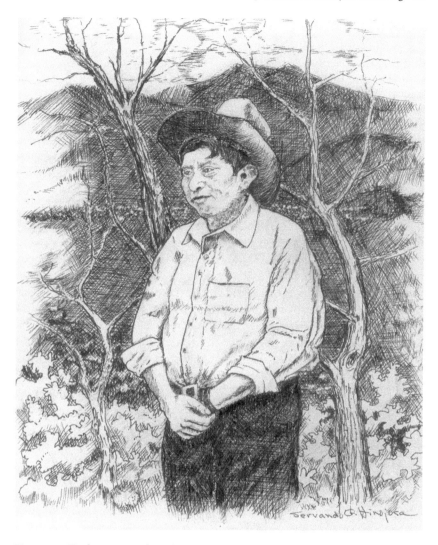

Figure 2.5. The bonesetter Alejandro, of Comalapa. Drawing courtesy of Servando G. Hinojosa.

could for them, but he would himself need help a couple of years later when he dislocated a finger. An old man came to treat him, he recalled. And while this may not have been the first bonesetter he interacted with, Alejandro probably noticed how the man worked on him and how his own injury improved. It improved so well, in fact, that not only was Alejandro able to resume working on his family plots, but he continued helping others with their injuries. Entering adulthood, he even began working as a primitivist painter, making him part of a still more unique local profession.

Alejandro's manual dexterity, then, developed in a context of healing, injury, and art. But unlike the bonesetter Bartolomé, he never received formal instruction. Alejandro only remembered seeing the diagram of a human skeleton at his school and being fascinated by how the bones looked. Since that time, he had come to know his way around injuries, and his hands developed a feel for the hidden structures of the body. One might say that, as with his paintings, which relied on faint guidelines to orient the eyes, his manual treatments rested on an innate knowledge of contours and masses directly perceivable by his hands.

Like other bonesetters, he usually performed his initial diagnostic manipulation in his home, when the clients could get there. And over many of these encounters he found that breaks, sprains, and dislocations could often swell in the same way. With a break, however, he said he could feel the broken bone under the skin and feel how the limb was limp. He would not feel this in the case of a sprain or dislocation. For the latter, he would apply the pomada Balsámico GMS, manipulate the area to move the bones as needed, and then wrap the injury. In fifteen days or so the client would be relieved of the pain, he said. Although dislocations might not seem as dangerous as fractures, for Alejandro they also required timely and diligent care because after fifteen to twenty days, the bones become harder to return to their position. Alejandro said that a "meat" even starts to grow in the articulation when left untreated, making the injury's treatment difficult.

He explained that clients came to him from throughout the region, even Guatemala City. According to Alejandro, these were people who did not want to go to hospitals and be placed in casts. But some individuals who took the clinical route wound up coming to him anyway. One such person was a man of about twenty-one who came to Alejandro's home late one morning. He had experienced a soccer injury at least two weeks before, and now appeared wearing bandages around his right shoulder and chest, and around his left knee. Describing his knee injury, he said that he had been to see a physical therapist, who had "popped" the bones of his knee four times, but he remained in pain.

Once Alejandro agreed to take a look, the young man handed him a commercial unguent called Dermolan, a product labeled for external veterinary use. The injured man had been applying it for its analgesic and anti-inflammatory properties; he did not say who had recommended it to him. Alejandro put the jar aside and seated the man across from him on a bench. He then had the client stretch out his injured leg, which Alejandro, who was seated, held on his own lap. Alejandro next lubricated the knee with the unguent. He then took the knee with both hands, pressed his thumbs directly below the kneecap, gently flexed the leg and extended it, then shook the leg while pulling it. Pausing a bit, he again squeezed the knee with both hands, bent the leg, and this time pushed the bent leg toward the client's torso. Alejandro seemed familiar with this maneuver.

Keeping a stoic face, the young man said his knee hurt whenever he exercised or when there was a change in the moon, like the night before. (There had been a full moon the night before, though, which is not usually known to exacerbate injuries.) He told us that he once had fractured his ankle and foot and had gone to a hospital, where he was X-rayed and put in a cast. But those clinicians did not do a good job, he said, since they left him with a protruding bone. Alejandro nodded upon hearing this familiar story.

Nearing the end of the treatment, Alejandro applied more unguent to the man's knee and wrapped it in a cloth. He recommended that the man massage his knee with the unguent every night. The Dermolan feels hot, Alejandro said, and it stimulates the injured area. Most people here know that heat is needed especially for dislocations, because cold *aire* can enter the joint and worsen the injury. As I discuss later in this chapter, aires can really complicate injuries, and bonesetters try to guard against them, which is not always easy. Alejandro had told me on an earlier occasion that he recommended performing massage treatments in the *tuj* in order to work in the hot and humid air there. He would have probably wanted to use the sweat bath for this client.[9]

Rolling his pant leg back down, the young man offered Alejandro a one-Quetzal note, even though Alejandro had not asked for anything. Pleased to see Alejandro finally accept it, the young man then said that he had gone earlier with another local bonesetter, Tonia, but the "cure" did not last. This made Alejandro his third choice to treat his injury, following the physical therapist and the first bonesetter. Together with his description of how he, to deal with yet another injury, also went to a hospital, a sense emerged that this young man had had unsatisfying experiences with a variety of providers, from clinicians to bonesetters. For the time being at least, he seemed happy with how Alejandro handled him. It was hard to picture another care provider lifting and pushing the young man's limb the way Alejandro did.

This was not the first time that Alejandro assisted someone who had been to other caregivers first, though he would probably have preferred to be first. Alejandro was well aware that such debilitating injuries could not wait: they could spell disaster for a breadwinner's ability to work. Simply put, it makes no sense harboring grudges about the order in which one is visited; the stakes are too high. By making himself available to others like this, without judgment, even when it meant soldiering through his own bodily pains and walking long distances across town, he earned a great deal of respect. His hands were stilled at age fifty-two at the San Juan de Dios Hospital in Guatemala City, where he passed with his wife at his side. A year later, when the granddaughter of another local bonesetter recalled Alejandro, she said, "He was the best bonesetter of Comalapa."

Rómulo

Although he did not know it at the time, when Rómulo was twelve years old he would treat someone in a way that would set his own path in bonesetting into motion. He was in the forest working with his father and brother-in-law. They felled a tree and then set about cutting off its branches. But just as the brother-in-law was cutting a limb, he slipped and fell. Rómulo says that the man "bent" his right foot, swinging it outward. They were ten kilometers from town and the man could not stand up, much less walk. That is when the brother-in-law told Rómulo, "Something tells me that you can fix me." Feeling he should act quickly, Rómulo resolved to do what he could. He told the man to hold on to something. Rómulo straightened out the man's foot at the ankle, then placed a stick against the foot and ankle. He then wrapped it all together with a T-shirt. They walked home that day, even though it was slow going. By the next day, says Rómulo, his brother-in-law showed pronounced recovery and he was already telling people about how Rómulo treated him. Things were never the same after this.

When he first started treating people, they would want to know right away if they had a fracture or a dislocation. So he had to let his hands reveal this to him. He says, "I began to probe, you could say, what is a bone, what is a fracture, and what is a deviation in the bones, what is a dislocation." As part of this process, Rómulo explains, "you have to make a little effort, pull on things a bit, reach the point on the bone where it's broken, because you can't do it just by pressing, because it won't reach—that's impossible. You have to give it a little tug, and move it just right to get it into its position, you know." It takes effort to find not just where the bone is

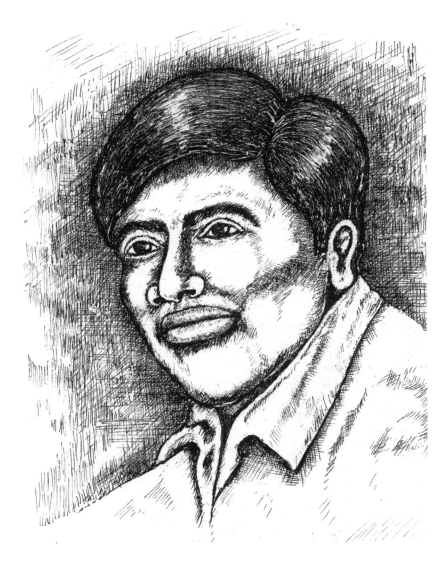

Figure 2.6. The bonesetter Rómulo, of Comalapa. Drawing courtesy of Servando G. Hinojosa.

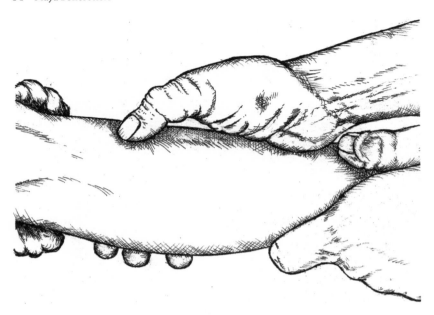

Figure 2.7. Rómulo presses his fingers onto the injured lower leg of his son. Drawing courtesy of Servando G. Hinojosa.

broken, but how the individual broken ends are positioned. Then come the pressing and pulling needed to realign the overall bone.

There is a lot his hands can detect even when there is no fracture or dislocation. When his son tells him he hurt himself in soccer practice a week ago, Rómulo sits the boy in front of him and takes a look at his left shin. He palpates the injured shin, then applies alcohol to the area. After a thorough rubbing he says, "Look at how swollen it is. It really looks swollen; see, it looks really purple; this here's the bone that's, that's . . ." Rómulo's words fade as his hands focus in on the front of the shin. As he pushes down with his thumb, he distinguishes the fleshy part of the front of the shin from the area where the tibia can be felt just beneath the skin. He remarks, "This is what is . . . see, where the bone is, yeah. It's a blow to the bone; it's the bone that got inflamed." Pointing to where different kinds of injuries occur on the lower leg, he says, "Here (would be) the blow to the muscle; here (would be) the blow to the bone; see, there it is, see." He continues pressing his thumb into the swollen part of the shin, confirming that the bone did not break: "No, no, it didn't break; it was only just a blow; the bone has a *chichón* [i.e., localized swelling], yes."

Rómulo then applies Balsámico GMS to the entire lower leg, commenting, "You know that you have to apply massage and pressure so that it, so that it goes down, let's say. It's, it's a swelling of the bone, yes, you have to apply massage and pressure." The area hurts, but luckily, his son's knee was not affected. "No, it wasn't affected—it was just the swelling. Yes, if that's from the bone it's really hard for it to subside, because the bone swells up. Yes, yes, it's the very bone, it isn't the skin but the very bone that swells up, yup." Rubbing his two thumbs on the boy's shin, he recalls how temperature changes can also be felt around injuries, saying, "You can feel the temperature. Sometimes when they have been hit really hard, the blood doesn't flow evenly, you can feel, let's say, that the temperature is very very, uh, how do you say it, very lukewarm; it isn't normal, so to speak. The, the body's heat, since the body has a certain heat, uh, normal heat, you know, right, but sometimes the body gets very, uh, freezing freezing cold. And that's because the blood as a whole isn't, isn't functioning well, yes."

Here he echoes the general idea, held by bonesetters, that injuries should be either kept warm or actively heated. Alejandro used Cofal and Dermolan to heat and stimulate injured areas, and Paulino used Mejoral and *calamentina* (pine resin; var. *trementina*) to do this.

How the heat is applied, though, depends on a couple of things. If the injury site shows a lot of inflammation, Rómulo recommends applying hot compresses of vinegar or of water in which the tip of an avocado branch has been boiled. The steam from the avocado decoction can also be directed at the injury. If a few days have passed since the person suffered his fracture, and the injury looks *morado* (bruised), Rómulo will also first apply a plant steam to the injury site. For this he might use steam from water boiled with either cypress, eucalyptus, or the tips of avocado or oak branches. He does this to heat up the *venas*, a term usually glossed as "veins" but here referring both to vascular pathways and connective tissue. The steam heats the venas, improves circulation, and makes the muscle more supple, allowing Rómulo to massage the area. If his clients do not believe in using these plants, though, he tells them to go and ask a physician for medication, showing how he is responsive to some clients' preference for commercial drugs. But by the time he sends them off, Rómulo says, he has already manually treated them.

His son's case shows how he normally does his diagnostic manipulation *en seco* (dry), at first. After he detects where the injury is, he then uses rubbing alcohol to ease the pain. An application of Balsámico GMS then fur-

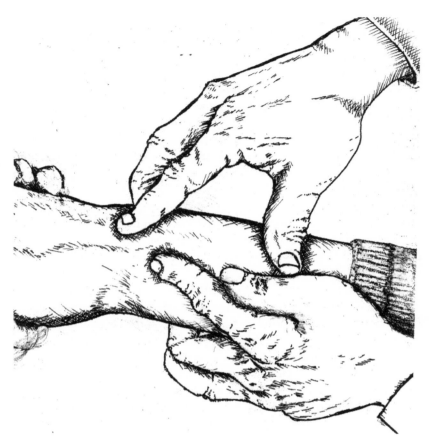

Figure 2.8. Rómulo points to the injured part of his son's lower leg. Drawing courtesy of Servando G. Hinojosa.

ther helps with the pain and lubricates the area for a massage. Rómulo is specific about what these two commercial products do: "The alcohol, first, it's that the alcohol penetrates and makes tender the, the body, and it acts to, as if it were something like an anesthesia. And now we can talk about the pomada, it's so that the, it calms the pain of the blow that, that is felt, it dissolves the injury of the muscle, you might say." So he uses a pomada-lubricant to ease the pain and dissolve the muscular injury, but only after detecting where the fracture is, or where, as he puts it, the venas were *estiradas* (stretched). He moves the bones after applying the pomada. Rómulo binds the boy's leg with an elastic bandage and says, "That's all that needs to be done, apply massage and pressure to him so that the bone, let's say, will reverse its inflammation." The boy will need a few more treatments: "Yes, that has to be done to him two or three times so that that . . . will return to normal, yup. Otherwise [the injury] can't, can't shrink all by itself. But we don't really know how it really is, we just, just found out [after all] that the kid was injured."

But whether he is treating a family member or a neighbor, in each case he invokes a higher power. Rómulo says, "I communicate with my Heavenly father . . . in order to do this work." As an *evangélico*, Rómulo's faith plays a role in his commitment to helping others. Despite his essentially pragmatic approach to treatment, he tells his clients that if they believe they will be cured, they will be cured, and if they do not believe, they will not be cured. His conviction about the source of his abilities aligns with his evangélico beliefs in affirming the healing power of God. But interestingly, in recognizing his conferred healing gifts, he echoes the way many traditionalist Mayas also identify the divine as the source of their healing gifts. This speaks to a larger discussion of how many evangélico Mayas exhibit practices traceable to preconversion belief structures.

On a more immediate level, though, Rómulo relies on his hands and on his past experience to guide his work. During the initial palpation, his hands read the signs of the body and guide him in how to pull and press on the injured area. Experience has taught him that after a fracture is first aligned and stabilized, it should not be moved for two or three days. It must remain at rest, *en reposo*, to let the mending begin. After this initial treatment, every three days the fracture site has to be unwrapped and carefully checked. "It has to be checked. If (the fracture) doesn't come out of place, it's because it's grabbing together, grabbing together. But it has to be checked, because without this inspection (the bone) can slip out of alignment again and the person winds up crippled." He must be certain that the fracture alignment is holding before he rewraps the site. About a month after the treatments have begun, if there is no movement at the ends of the bone, Rómulo tells her or him to start moving the limb. He has come to recommend this step "so that the tendons don't remain stiff." If the tendons stay stiff, the treatment will be useless. The injured body part should start moving at this point because, he says, "all the body's movements should be resumed until the movement returns to normal."

The process can take longer with fractures that are more challenging in general, such as femur fractures. These are the most difficult to treat, Rómulo says, because the thigh is so *carnoso* (meaty). Bandaging it is one problem. One has to find a satisfactory way of wrapping the thigh, he says, because if you place too much bandaging, it will swell. Keeping the fractured femur aligned is another issue. The leg has to be immobilized from the hip all the way to the foot, with the foot itself immobilized to keep it from turning and undoing the alignment in the thigh. According to Rómulo, this kind of fracture takes about three months to heal, if all goes well. But things do not always go well.

When Rómulo has faced major fractures such as this, he has often had to deal with more than just the bone. Some people seek his help but do not really cooperate with him, and when they do not cooperate with him the treatment process can get muddled. He gives the example of a client from Xetonur village. The man broke a femur when a load of grass fell on him. Then, according to Rómulo, three people tried to treat him, but because they said he had a dislocation and not a fracture, they did not treat him properly. By the time the injured man was brought to Rómulo, more than a month had passed. He saw that not only was the man's femur fractured, but the proximal end of the broken femur was pressing against the skin on the outer side of the thigh. Rómulo told the man that he had a fracture. It was a bad break, said the bonesetter, because the femur was broken in two places, and the separated middle section had an additional large separated chip along the bottom. Moreover, the breaks were angled, not perpendicular to the shaft. This kind of fracture, Rómulo tells me, slips easily even after it has been aligned.

The injured man would not accept the diagnosis, though. When he said he did not believe Rómulo, the latter suggested the man go and get an X-ray. Hearing this, the man decided to trust Rómulo and submit to treatment. The first time Rómulo manipulated the man's leg, it really hurt the client. Rómulo says the chip that had separated from the middle bone fragment is what gave him trouble. For a month Rómulo treated the man every three days, but every time he would examine him he found that the ends of the bone had moved. Apparently, the man kept undoing the immobilization and was moving too much. Rómulo suspected that the man was getting anxious, and this was getting the bones out of line. Frustrated at what he was seeing, Rómulo told the man he would treat him only once more. At this, the man finally agreed to stop moving his leg and as a result was cured. This episode showed Rómulo that the client has to be part of the solution: "One has to do his part," Rómulo says, stressing the need for cooperation. Today, the injured man in question can walk. It was a tough case and the final alignment was not perfect, but, as Rómulo says, "sometimes a little deviation remains, but one can only do so much."

This case strained Rómulo's patience, but another case recently tested his physical resourcefulness. Rómulo describes how a man had fallen into a gorge two days earlier and had broken four ribs. When this first happened, Rómulo was called out to the man's village to treat him. The man was in a lot of pain and could neither lie nor sit down. When Rómulo would touch the man's ribs, he not only felt the breaks but also could hear the rib tips moving against each other. Sensing that the ribs were fractured, as confirmed by the crepitus, he knew he would have to pull them back into place somehow.

Since he could not grasp the ribs directly, he used a suction technique. He rubbed the skin with alcohol as he usually did, then placed a lit candle on a coin and placed the coin on the skin. He then put a glass over the candle and let it burn out, creating a vacuum. With the glass firmly attached to the skin over the ribs, he pulled the cup upward with a twisting motion, moving the ribs along with the skin. Rómulo says the alcohol and the gas it contains are what pulls the skin. But if the skin is too wet with alcohol sometimes the alcohol ignites, even if this was not intended. This technique is useful, then, for rib fractures in which you cannot directly grab the skin. He also recommends using this method, elsewhere known as *ventosas* (cupping), where the ribs meet the sternum. After applying the glasses to the injured man, Rómulo then wrapped a six-inch-wide bandage several times around his chest, "to restrain, contain" the ribs. Today was the man's third treatment, and he will receive six or seven treatments in all. But he is already doing better, says Rómulo. He can now lie down.

Rómulo has learned many lessons through such experiences. Whether he is facing emotional pushback from a client or anatomical barriers to treatment, he has needed to think things through before taking the next step. Now forty-seven, he can look back at a three-decade career in bonesetting and feel he has been helpful. His biggest contentment comes from knowing that "nearly all" (as he puts it) who have come to him have turned out well.

Bodies, Age, and Self-Treatment

To even begin to show the skill and resourcefulness that they put to work, bonesetters have to know a lot about how bodies are built. But it is not enough to have working knowledge of the musculoskeletal frame. As Tomás points out, "There's something else: the age of the person matters," as bodies heal differently according to how old the injured person is. Once they begin attending injuries, bonesetters find out that the younger the person, the more rapidly he or she heals, as Tiv bonesetters of Nigeria have also noted (Nyityo 1990–1991–1992:39). And because younger people's bones mend much faster than those of older people, according to Tomás and Rómulo, they need to be treated sooner after an injury, before the breaks ossify. This is one more way that bonesetters have to engage differently with different kinds of bodies.

After attending to the injuries of people from two months to eighty years of age, Tomás is attuned to age-based differences. In general, he says, kids ten and under might take fifteen to twenty days, or fewer, to recover from many injuries. People aged thirty to forty are also strong, and "they get cured quickly." But for people ages sixty to eighty, it is a different story. "It's hard for them to join," Tomás says of their bones' ability to recover from fractures. These people might break bones in their thighs, shins, hips, or backs, and the healing really takes longer. He reasons that they do not respond well to treatment because their bodies lack vitamins or because their bodies simply "no longer grow." Because of their advanced age, he finds he has to treat them slowly and calmly, taking much more time. In the end their delicate state and patchy progress take a toll on him, too. In his words, "sometimes I really start to suffer along with them . . . it feels slow."

Rómulo agrees that children heal more rapidly and that their recovery process is much better. He states that children and adults can usually recover from fractures in two to three months because they are at an age "when they still have strength." On the other hand, older people take longer, perhaps four to five months, to recover from fractures because "their bones no longer show growth." An older person's fracture can be corrected, he contends, but only after a longer period. This is not entirely good news for children, though, because rapid healing has its drawbacks. Rómulo says that if a child's broken bone is "very compacted," "it can no longer be fixed because the bone grows rapidly. A child has to be treated more promptly." With the smaller window of opportunity for treating a child before the injury resists repair, bonesetters have to be vigilant. Kids routinely break their arms, legs, shoulders, clavicles, and ribs, Rómulo states. And why are they so prone to injury? He chuckles. "Kids are more naughty and *traviesos* [naughtily active] than us grown-ups."

Soccer players, meanwhile, present their own set of problems. Because of their frequent injuries and their youth, their teammates or relatives usually take them right away to bonesetters when they take a hit. The bonesetter Lupito comments, "Those who come [to me] the most are the boys, because they play *fútbol*. If it's not the foot, it's the hand." Local

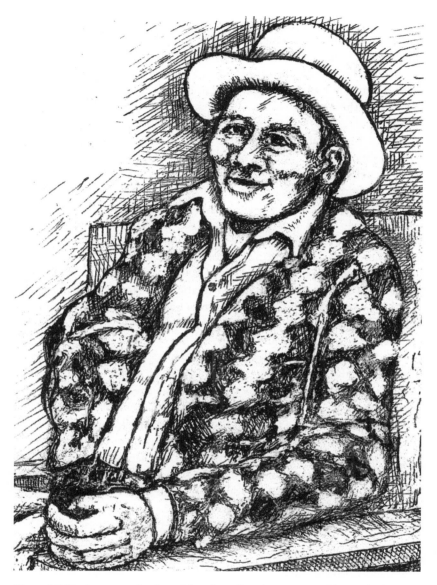

Figure 2.9. The bonesetter Lupito, of Comalapa. Drawing courtesy of Servando G. Hinojosa.

bonesetters have even had to treat injured players right on the pitch during matches. Alejandro remembered going to a match as a spectator and then getting called in to treat an injured player.

Having a feel for bodies of different ages is one part of the bonesetters' suite of skills, but as part of their larger approach to treatment they also expect that their clients will participate in their own care. Bonesetters encourage their clients to perform some follow-up self-treatment, simple as it may be. They might recommend exercises to keep body parts stable or to keep them moving. Or they might recommend some purchases at the pharmacy. Lupito regularly urges his clients to couple the care he gives them with additional treatments at home. For example, while he treats a man whose thumb got bent backwards in a fall, he tells him that when he gets home he should apply hot water to it. Using his own thumb, Lupito then shows him how he should practice flexing the tip of his thumb. Similarly, when he finishes treating a young woman who has injured the tendons of her left ring finger, he tells her, "You have to do exercises." He curls his own fingers a few times in demonstration. Moreover, she will need to heat her hand to do this. "When it's gotten hot with water, you need to do the exercise, and then this will normalize. Here, here is where you need to do this," Lupito explains, singling out her finger joints.

Like Lupito, Tomás knows his clients cannot visit him every day, so he offers some advice for the interim. As he wraps up a visit to a woman with severely sprained ankles, he recommends that she get a device called a *tobillero*. Available at the pharmacy, this ankle brace will fit around the top, bottom, and back of the foot and provide good support. Devices such as these work well, Tomás says, so long as they are not put on so tightly that they impede circulation. But wearing this will not mean she can put her full weight on her feet. Tomás reminds her that she will have to cut back on her walking and work for the duration of her treatment. The last thing he wants is for her to reinjure her ankles.

A speedier recovery is also on the mind of the bonesetter Tonia when she treats a fracture. According to the parents of a girl who broke her wrist by falling into a trench and who was treated by Tonia, this bonesetter offered them advice throughout the treatment. Tonia first placed stiff cardboard on the girl's right wrist for three days, then she affixed a homemade cast to the injury. This stayed on for three weeks. During this time the girl developed a large swelling, so Tonia told her parents to buy a certain anti-inflammatory drug that she said was "good for fractures." They bought the drug and gave it to the girl, whose swelling then subsided. Once Tonia removed the cast and wrapped the wrist in a bandage, she told the family that the girl had to do hand exercises. She showed the girl how to clench her fist, and then told her she had to keep trying to clench her right fist. At first the girl could not do it, but the more she tried it at home, the more movement and strength gradually returned. But while Tonia offered self-treatment recommendations in the context of solid cast immobilization, solid casting is itself rare in Maya bonesetting. Most bonesetters use removable immobilization devices, not casts, an important distinction between Maya and clinical approaches.

Immobilization without Casting

Casting is a technology that can interfere with hand-based healing, so bonesetters generally avoid it. Few Maya bonesetters apply casts to broken bones because to do so would prevent the bonesetter from checking the injury as it heals and adjusting it, if necessary. Immobilization using easily removable materials—cardboard, sticks, cloth, maguey cordage, and the like (Holland 1963:177)—has thus long been preferred over the use of solid plaster. To this list we can now add elastic bandages and even plywood. So when Maya bonesetters do decide to apply casts, they make every effort to first properly reduce the fracture before covering it (Cosminsky 1972:182). Those who do cast, moreover, see casting as but one way to immobilize an injury site, and not the only way.

One reason bonesetters avoid casts is that physicians routinely use them in care (often in conjunction with X-rays) that bonesetters consider to be poor. According to bonesetters, physicians frequently mishandle fractures by not reducing them properly and then immobilizing them, causing pain or deformity. The bonesetter Tomás offers his view of how physicians treat and cast fractures: "Well, some [physicians] do know how to fix them, and there's some who, right when a patient arrives at the hospital, go, 'Let's see what you got,' and just bind [cast] him up and 'That's it, get out, out, out, out.' Then those people come to me; they've been made to suffer. That's what they do in the hospitals."

Guatemalan bonesetters generally have such a negative view of casting that if an injured person with a cast goes to a bonesetter, the bonesetter will often remove the cast to treat the injury. One example was related by researcher-client McMahon in 1994, when he took his fractured right fibula (broken near the ankle) to a hospital in Guatemala City, where it was X-rayed and casted. When the pain continued, he went to a bonesetter in San Pedro La Laguna. The bonesetter removed McMahon's cast and manipulated his ankle and foot over two consecutive days (McMahon 1994: 164). The experience left McMahon with a fully healed bone, as shown in a later X-ray, and with the confirmation that the Guatemalan medical sector places undue emphasis on casting as a therapeutic tool.

As in other parts of Guatemala, in Comalapa it is not unusual for bonesetters to be approached by people who have been fitted with a cast, and by most accounts these people are in bad shape. When they have to, most local bonesetters will remove a cast to reach an injured limb. But in many cases, sufferers will come to bonesetters having already removed their casts. Rómulo describes visits from people who have been in a cast for three or four months and who do not feel they are getting well. He often finds that their fractures have not healed or have not healed correctly. There is not much that can be done with fractures that have already knitted, but, he says, the fracture "can be corrected when the bone hasn't grown too much." This, he contends, is more often the case with older persons than with children. Alejandro likewise tells me that people have removed their own casts and then come to him. These reports suggest not only that many traumatic injuries receive clinical treatment that the injured find unsatisfactory, but also that some bonesetters in Comalapa have learned to refrain from removing casts themselves. In order to avoid problems with physicians, in fact, Tomás has the person wearing the cast remove the cast himself because otherwise, he says, "I make a big mistake." He risks getting singled out by physicians for undoing their work.[10] Only after the plaster appliance comes off will Tomás palpate the injury, at which point he often finds "the bone is still broken, it didn't come out well"; "[the bones] are just not in the right condition, you know." He then has to "arrange" the bones for what he hopes will be the last time, and decide how to immobilize the site.

While some bonesetters use solid immobilization, the vast majority does not, and the public does not associate bonesetters with casting. One more often hears about Maya bonesetters *removing* hard casts than applying them. Removable materials, in contrast, allow the bonesetters to monitor and remanipulate the injury sites as needed (see Lambert 1995: 97–98). Be that as it may, one Comalapa bonesetter, Tonia, has been known to make hard casts, as mentioned earlier. Although I met her only briefly and was not able to have long conversations with her, I heard many people talk about her over the years. The accounts did not usually reflect well on her. As for why she had a mixed reputation, I got the sense that not only did she dismiss some people's pain reports and say they were not injured, but she used hard casting in conjunction with other care. And because many of her clients' outcomes were not good, those clients often recalled her casting practice in ways that faulted her overall skill set.[11]

Her approach to bonesetting is unusual not only because she uses hard casts, but because of the form they take and how she came to use them. While she sometimes makes splints from pieces of stiff cardboard, she is more known for preparing casts made from a hardening mixture of flour and egg whites, as a local physician has confirmed (Icú Perén 1990:57). Like other bonesetters, she knows that different kinds of fractures require different kinds of fixation and that heavy casting is not always needed. But if she feels that she has aligned a fracture well and it looks stable, she might cast it. Notably, this does not mean she will be unable to remanipulate the injury. According to another local physician whose patient had been one of Tonia's former clients, the cast that Tonia applied to her client was "removable." This would have let Tonia periodically check how the client's broken wrist was mending.

What is also noteworthy about her cast-making practice is that, according to a family whose child she treated, Tonia first learned about making casts in a dream. The dream, which she experienced after asking God how to help her patients, revealed how she was to make casts using flour, eggs, and cooking oil. Though it is unclear whether she made casts before she had this revelation (or whether her casts have always been removable), the fact that she makes casts is still quite unusual for a Comalapa bonesetter, especially since so many Comalapans dislike how clinicians use these devices. To the extent that local people have allowed her to cast them, it may be because her casts were revealed to her in a dream, an important vehicle of healing validation, and because some of the casts are removable and thus compatible with how local bonesetting works. Her frequent use of this technology remains the exception, though.

It is more often the case that bonesetters find themselves confronting casts applied by clinicians. When this happens, clients and bonesetters have found ways of working around hard casts, even having the patients remove them, or occasionally removing them themselves, when they think this is warranted. As one might expect, the bonesetters' tendency to remove casts irritates physicians to no end. What physicians find even more unsettling, though, is that some Maya bonesetters might have learned their skills by treating animals.

Early Learning from Animals

Interestingly, Maya and other bonesetters have been known to treat the injuries of animals from around the farm and household (Cosminsky 1972:182; Elliott 1981:253). This is not in and of itself surprising, given the rural base of their practice and their need for self-sufficiency. Nor is it surprising, perhaps, that many Guatemalan bonesetters began their work in this way. According to Icú Perén (1990:47), for example, some Comalapa Maya bonesetters said they began their practice by treating injured dogs, cows, horses, and cats. Similarly, Maya scholar Enrique Sam Colop wrote in a newspaper editorial in 2007 that a bonesetter from Cantel first learned his craft by treating his injured sheep (Sam Colop 2007). If a sheep broke its leg while he was out with it, he would set its leg with a splint made of tree bark. The man went on to gain a widespread reputation for treating people. He even treated Guatemalan football players and army paratroopers.

Reflecting a wider pattern of experience in Guatemala, the sole local bonesetter in Todos Santos Cuchumatán began his career by treating a dog's broken leg (Acevedo Ligorria 1986:82–84). But even though he began his work with animals (and though he was Ladino), this was less important to locals than the fact that he lived and worked in a town that bore a heavy burden of injury. His Mam Maya neighbors saw his skills as legitimate, however he may have attained them. Nonetheless, while these local residents may have played down the fact that he began his work by helping animals, this acceptance of bonesetters irrespective of their animal patients is not a generalizable feature of Maya communities, and certainly not in Comalapa.

Alejandro, for example, warned that if one has the gift of healing and one uses it on animals, the gift will be forfeited. He himself did not begin by treating animals, which might explain his disapproval of the practice. But not all would agree with him about losing the gift of healing if one treats animals. It is more likely the case that bonesetters who do not treat animals may be trying to limit the size of their overall clientele. The treating of animals seems to become an issue only when a given bonesetter treats people *in addition* to treating animals. The implication is that a bonesetter should treat people *or* animals, but not both. Alejandro's wife further explains that treating animals can affect a bonesetter's abilities. She says that the bonesetter Tonia's clients have been coming to see Alejandro, and then obliquely adds that since Tonia had supposedly started treating the fractures of dogs and piglets, she does not, or cannot, heal humans any more.

Whether Tonia actually treats animals, the insinuation that she does treat them is consonant with her reputation for having mixed success in treating people. Arturo, a Comalapan educator, raises a similar concern about another bonesetter. He says that there used to be a really famous bonesetter in Comalapa named Tulio, but people stopped going to see him. Apparently, one day Tulio tried to heal a dog. After curing an animal, Arturo says, a curer can no longer heal people. His hands lose their knowledge of human bones. Without going into specifics, Arturo explained that for a person such as Tulio to regain his ability to heal people, he would have to go through a certain "process."

Bonesetters might also avoid treating animals because of a question of status. As I will discuss in chapter 3, bonesetting is not considered a high-status activity in the region. Some bonesetters might therefore want to elevate their practice by distancing it from animal handling, which would also deflect some criticisms by physicians, at any rate. Other bonesetters might also want to encourage the idea that while their hands can connect with suffering bodies, they can connect only with *human* suffering bodies, not with bodies in general. Regardless of whether they want fewer clients or higher status, though, bonesetters express no consensus about taking on animals as patients. Treating animals remains an open question, and for those bonesetters who worry that their work with animals might reflect badly on them, it remains a somewhat sensitive subject.

A Word on Costs

Bonesetters do not like talking about what they charge for their work. From what I can ascertain, they normally accept from one to ten quetzals per treatment, with most payments around the middle of this range. While there is no agreement about what bonesetters should charge, they generally agree that they should not ask their clients for payment. Any exchange of money should be considered an *agradecimiento*, a gesture of thanks and not an obligation. Some clients might also leave some commercial products, for example, pomada, with their bonesetters after receiving treatment, and in a sense this might be considered part of the agradecimiento.

The degree to which bonesetters downplay or try to conceal the receipt of money surfaces on several occasions. When the time comes for clients to offer the bonesetters something, the bonesetters usually smile nervously and refuse to accept anything. It is only after the client prevails upon them to accept something that the bonesetter will take some quetzals into his hand. How much money actually changes hands following these ritualized refusals depends, of course, on the number of clients a bonesetter treats and what they can pay. There are no clear measures of how many clients bonesetters see per day, though, because each bonesetter's daily workload can vary dramatically. One late bonesetter in Comalapa would go days without seeing a client, whereas another one in the Lake Atitlán area sees upwards of twenty clients per day. These two individuals are outliers in this sense. Taking the daily workload fluctuations of other bonesetters into account, most individual bonesetters probably see an average of two or three clients a day. No matter how many people come to them, though, bonesetters are not supposed to seem overly interested in what they carry in their pockets.

While there operates an understanding that bonesetters will be paid for services delivered, the last thing that bonesetters want is to garner a money-hungry reputation. They do not want to be seen as profiteers. It is not unusual for bonesetting clients, and even bonesetters, to talk about bonesetters who charge far more than they should, even up to sixty or a hundred quetzals per treatment. Aside from letting people voice their disapproval of particular bonesetters, when people refer to bonesetters in this way their remarks probably also serve to informally discourage bonesetters from overcharging. Bonesetters are supposed to welcome with humility and even hesitation whatever people can offer them.[12] If they fail to do this and instead make money the driver of their work, the public can call their legitimacy into question.

An aversion to monetized transactions may be one mark of the bonesetter's legitimacy, and an important one at that, but there are others. Bonesetters are expected to be as attentive to the larger world in which injuries happen as they are expected to be inattentive to matters of payment. As someone who handles many suffering bodies, the bonesetter is constantly reminded of how larger natural forces act upon and through these bodies. Annual rainfall patterns and monthly lunar changes, for instance, can really make themselves felt in bodies. The bonesetter somatically witnesses the effects of these cycles in the aches, pains, and debilities people bring him, making knowledge of our earthly surroundings a big part of his work.

Bonesetters and the Natural Environment

Along with their hand-based intuition, bonesetters bring another asset to the healing craft: their knowledge of the natural environment. Much of the bonesetters' work speaks to the relationship between human bodies and changing natural phenomena, such as the rainy and dry seasons and lunar cycles.[13] Bonesetters are also wary of how other, less perceptible environmental agents likewise affect the body, moving through the spaces between bodies and into bodies themselves. When we consider the degree to which bonesetters pay attention to their natural surroundings, it becomes clear that the physicality of their role extends out to and includes an engagement with forces operating on a much larger scale. To be effective at their work, then, they must have close knowledge of the physical world they inhabit.

Bonesetters pay close attention to the changing seasons around them, for instance. In highland Guatemala, where seasonal changes consist of an alternating rainy season from May to October and a dry season from November to April, bonesetters can expect sizeable fluctuations in their caseload. Bonesetters report that during the rainy season, for instance, as trails turn muddy, people run a higher risk of slipping and falling, especially if the trails are steep or if one is carrying a heavy load. Maneuvering through these trails in the dark, as many must, is especially hazardous. These conditions result in a higher incidence of sprains and other falling injuries, true also for children. During the dry season, on the other hand, the problem with another environmental reality intensifies.

As many indigenous Guatemalans are aware, something called *aires* can imperil the body, especially when the weather is cold and dry. Aires are types of air or gaseous entities considered harmful to the body (Tedlock 1987:1074; Wisdom 1940:56). They are usually thought of as media or vehicles of harm, even supernatural harm (Bricker et al. 1998:12, 247; García et al. 1999:247; Lipp 1991:158; Reina 1962:29). But what worries bonesetters the most about aires is how they are said to penetrate the body to bad effect, especially because of their cold temperature valence. Because of their cold quality, aires are said to worsen pain and swelling in sites of bodily injury. This makes bonesetters careful to keep injured areas warm. And because they see so many cases of people worsening their injuries by carelessly exposing themselves to aires, bonesetters caution that the body should always be shielded from aires and their coldness. The best way to do this when it is cold outside is simply to stay home and stay warm, but this is not an option for most people. Since people have to be out and about when cold aires are a problem, they are repeatedly advised to wear plenty of warm clothing. To do otherwise puts healthy bodies at risk and can make it harder to deal with injured bodies.

The cold nature of aires presents certain considerations for the treatment of injuries, compelling bonesetters to use both hot products and hot environments when treating people. To counteract the cold, Emilio and other bonesetters make sure to use hot water when massaging injured bodies. For Emilio, the ideal place to do these massages is the *tuj*, or the family *temascal*, or sweat bath, found in many Comalapan homes. The bonesetter Alejandro also recommends massaging in the tuj because of its hot and humid interior, something echoed by Bartolomé. The elderly Bartolomé says that the tuj is especially good for treating injuries that show swelling, because swellings are inherently cold. Emilio adds that once he massages and heats the body, it is best to apply a layer of cotton and then a bandage to the injury so that aire does not enter, "para sostener el calor" (in order to maintain the heat). Meanwhile, Rómulo insists that injuries should be placed only in hot water, never cold. This is because the injuries can become *reumáticos*, more inflamed and painful, if they are placed rapidly in cold water. It is better to treat them with hot water.

The way bonesetters talk about the products they use reflects their ongoing concern with the cold and its attendant pain and swelling, especially in postinjury treatment. For instance, Alejandro says that the commercial pomada Cofal is good at "taking out the *frío* [cold]," as is garlic. Another bonesetter, Paulino, applies a pine resin he calls *calamentina* (Sp. *trementina*, Kaq. *q'ol*) to the injury to heat the area and deflect aires. This treatment keeps aires from entering the body, he says, which would otherwise cause pain. Emilio rubs alcohol onto injury sites, but then promptly applies the product Pomada GMS, "para que no se entre el aire, porque con el aire se hincha, al rato menos" (so that aire doesn't get in because with aire, [the injury] swells in moments). Then he affixes a bandage to insulate the area. For Rómulo, heated vinegar works great on swollen and painful injuries because vinegar treats the exact bodily tissues that aires target. While he agrees that "when one is injured, the *poros* open up, and *aire* enters the body," he points out that when aire enters the body it penetrates especially the *venas* and *tendones*, making them swell. This swelling then causes the affected muscles to part into two bunches or groups, which in turn produces pain. But heated vinegar ostensibly relaxes the muscles by reducing the swelling of the venas and tendones, says Rómulo, thus relieving the pain.

Generally, after treating a person's injury, bonesetters try to keep the

injured area warm and protected from aires. To preserve the hot benefits of the treatment, they recommend covering the injury with cotton
and bandages and then with immobilizing materials, if needed. They must
keep the area warm because some injuries, such as dislocations, are especially vulnerable to cold aires. Alejandro says that when dislocations swell,
cold aires are often to blame. That this happens a lot does not surprise
him, because so many people go around exposed to the cold. In some cases
of dislocation, Alejandro takes an additional step to shield against aires.
After manipulating the area, he makes a "tortilla" out of moist clay and
packs it onto the injury. This, together with a bandage layered on top,
works to keep out the aires and their coldness. To spot-heat injury sites,
Comalapa Kaqchikel bonesetters also use commercial salves, Vaseline, or
even *sebo de res* (beef fat), available from butchers (Icú Perén 1990:55).

Bonesetters seem to put into practice their views of an interchange of
aire between the body and the environment, and these interchanges can
take different forms. In one form, as Alejandro explains, when one feels
lots of gas in the intestines, aire is the problem. This happens when one is
hungry but does not eat, in which case aire will enter the intestines and
cause turmoil, to the point that it *da vuelta* (churns). To treat this, Alejandro positions the sufferer on all fours and massages his or her abdomen,
trying to move the aire out rectally. Then, with the sufferer lying on his
or her back, he continues massaging the abdomen and places a cloth bag
filled with hot ashes on the person's abdomen, to be worn overnight. His
concerns about intestinal aires call to mind how among K'iche' Mayas,
swimming in a cold river can cause water to penetrate the skin and enter
the stomach, producing gas and flatulence, symptoms associated with still
other cold afflictions (Tedlock 1987:1074).

Infusions of aire into the body can also take other, more severe, forms
in Comalapa. A midwife reports that the stomach of a person with fright
sickness can fill with aire, causing inflammation and discomfort. It must
be treated ritually. In another case, Emilio recounts that he was once hit
by a gust of aire that knocked him to the ground. He was then taken with
fever. Following this, something that he calls a "nerve paralysis" swept
over the left side of his body, whereupon Encarnación, another bonesetter,
was called to treat him. Following the treatment, Encarnación made sure
to leave Emilio covered up in a blanket so that the aire would not penetrate
him again and worsen him (see also García et al. 1999:43). The severity of
this case recalls Charles Wisdom's (1940) description of Chorti' Maya massagers and "surgeons" in eastern Guatemala. He reported that healers in
this group tried to push *aigres* (aires) out of the body either by massaging

the body in the direction of a limb or extremity or by moving the hands above the body in like fashion (1940:355). In some cases, aigres trapped in the body could cause great pain. When this happened, the Chorti' surgeon would use a small flint knife to "open the flesh to permit an *aigre* to escape" (356), cutting about half an inch deep. The pain would continue until the aigre was released.

Fortunately, cold aires present more modest risks for most people's bodies. On one chilly Comalapan afternoon, for example, after massaging my back with the pomada Cofal, Alejandro cautions me to put on another sweater if I plan to continue doing errands outside that day, so that my back will not get cold. And the reason my back was hurting in the first place? My back might have felt *frío* (cold) from when I drove in from another town earlier that day. As a general rule, the avoidance of cold also extends to the bonesetter himself. Alejandro cautions that one must not handle cold water when one is applying emollients such as Pomada GMS, or the massager can endanger his own arms with excessive cold. Emilio has firsthand experience of this. Suffering from chronic arm pain, he suspects that the pain comes from his having washed in cold water, but he does not say when he did this.

For all the precautions one might take, cold aires can still get to people, especially the ailing and the elderly. Bartolomé speaks of the debilities that come with his age, but stresses that he suffers cold, cramping leg pains due to the cold. He shows me how he wraps his legs all the way down to his ankles, just to dull the cold in his knees a little bit. When the rains come, it feels particularly cold, and his legs bear the brunt. The cold also afflicts Pascual, another elderly man, to the point that he regularly places leaves of *may* (*Kaq.*; green tobacco) on his legs to alleviate feelings of pain and coldness. He often asks me to bring him leaves from the tobacco plant growing in my garden. To use them, he places the fresh leaves directly on his bare lower legs, wraps a plastic sheeting around them, and then wears socks over the sheeting. He shows me that when the leaves have done their job heating him, they become dry and brittle, and need replacing.[14]

These men know that the pains that cold aires bring are not limited to the dry months of the year, however. While aires are more of a problem during the dry season, when it is rather cold outdoors, vulnerability to aires also occurs cyclically on a daily basis. The early morning and evening hours, being comparatively cold, harbor more dangers for people with injuries or with aging-related infirmities. People develop their own strategies for minimizing their exposure to daily aires and coldness, such as by washing clothes or bathing only during the warmest hours of the afternoon, or by bathing in a tuj and bundling up immediately afterward.

To hear it from Kaqchikels in Comalapa, it is clear that injuries and pains are of a cold character and that these can get exacerbated by aires, also of a cold character, such that shielding the body and injuries from the cold makes sense. It also makes sense for bonesetters to employ heat and avoid cold in their treatments, whether in the healing environment or in the substances they use. The temperature valence picture is not so uniform in the larger Maya area, though. Among Tzeltal and Tzotzil Mayas of Chiapas, for instance, different kinds of bodily injuries and pains are considered to have a hot, not cold, temperature valence. These conditions run the risk of "attracting" cold qualities, however, which would worsen them. An important way to block the cold is to use the local sweat bath, which warms the blood and keeps heat in the body (Groark 1997:64–65). Other researchers in highland Chiapas likewise point to a local treatment system at some variance with highland Guatemala's. Elois Ann Berlin and Brent Berlin (1996:64–65) report that localized swellings are treated with a "cold virtue therapy" and that injuries ranging from fractures to sprains are dealt with using both warm and cold plants. Temperature valence–based systems thus operate in the different regions, though not identically.

With their knowledge of the wet and dry seasons, and of the action of aires, Guatemala Maya bonesetters often have to adjust their work in tandem with their changing surroundings. But just as bonesetters recognize interaffect between the body and aires, they also view the body as highly vulnerable to the moon's influence. Alejandro explains that the phase of the moon affects the strength of the body. When the moon is full, and thus stronger, so, too, is the body stronger. The body becomes more resistant during this lunar phase. It can resist injury better and will not bleed excessively if cut. However, during the new moon, the moon's state of weakness becomes shared by the body. People must be careful because their bodies become more prone to accident and injury at this time. If they cut themselves, they might even bleed more. A midwife tells me that a woman who delivers during a new moon will release more birth fluid. Alejandro says that during the new moon, not only does he feel more back pain, but he notices his leg falling asleep more often (Hinojosa 2002:36n2).

It is not clear whether the moon directly conveys its changed states to the human body, but both bodies manifest concurrent changes, resulting in the more delicate bodily states often linked to mishaps and injury.

Comalapan Maya bonesetters and Comalapans generally recognize as well that the new moon contributes a broad-spectrum debility to all bodies in nature, from trees, to crops, to animals and children. Conversely, the full moon has a strengthening effect on all bodies. In this scheme, the most auspicious time to conceive a child is during the full moon, so that the child will grow up strong, hardworking, and intelligent. Sometimes it is said that changes in the body occur because of a *change* in the moon, as when the moon is in the process of reaching full invisibility or full visibility. In this case, too, bonesetters foreground the body's empathy with the lunar cycle. As body specialists, it is the bonesetters' job to understand how the body interacts with other aspects of nature and how this can cause injury and infirmity. The attribution of these and other effects to the moon is also found in other parts of Mesoamerica (Lipp 1991:18, 60; Wisdom 1940:299).

Much of the bonesetter's work speaks to the relationship between human bodies and other aspects of the natural world, particularly the seasons, with their variable aires, and the moon. To attend effectively to the suffering body, then, the Comalapan bonesetter has to discern how the cycles connected to these entities interact with the body's states of strength. Doing this, his hands can detect the body's injuries and begin alleviating them when the time comes. With the bonesetters' concern for the body's well-being situated in a world of flux, it is clear that the physicality of their role extends out to and includes an engagement with natural phenomena. But the approach taken by bonesetters of other places suggests that other forces are at work in injured bodies and in those who treat them. These specialists recognize a greater role for the supernatural in injury diagnosis and treatment, to the point that they exhibit an uncharacteristically ritualized view of bones and of themselves. The next chapter discusses one ritualized form of bonesetting that is thriving in two communities.

CHAPTER 3

Sacred Forms of Maya Bonesetting

Bonesetting in San Pedro La Laguna and San Juan La Laguna

One of the most arresting sights I have seen in Guatemala is happening on the shore of Lake Atitlán, where the town of San Pedro La Laguna meets the water. It is 1998, and I am watching a group of men struggling to unload a small boat moored to a private dock. With bystanders urging everyone to keep steady, the boat dips and rocks precariously as the men step onto the weathered platform. Once they move onto the dock's uneven planks, though, they cannot set their load down for even a moment. They have to keep moving because their cargo is a man in a makeshift stretcher, and the four men bearing his weight are here to deliver him to one of the town's Maya bonesetters.

The boat that brings this man to San Pedro La Laguna is one of many that normally carry produce and passengers around the lake and that, like the lake itself, has now been pressed into providing other kinds of services. The growing number of transports such as this one is part of a shift locals have seen toward more export-oriented agriculture and tourism over the last forty years, one driving changes that are now deeply enmeshed with local economies. But even though these new income streams have made many towns around Lake Atitlán more dependent on shifting commodity prices and foreign currency valuations, inhabitants of San Pedro La Laguna and its neighbor San Juan La Laguna have not handed complete control of their lives over to outsiders. They still try to meet whatever needs they can locally, including treating themselves when they get injured. And for this, locals rely on the area's Tz'utujiil Maya bonesetters.

Like the people arriving on the boat, local people are intensely aware of the bonesetters who live and work here. They also know that the bonesetters' reputations extend to the far edges of the country, something that brings in the occasional care-seeker from El Salvador or Mexico. Most of those who come are Guatemalan, though, and in one way or another they have heard that local curers use a unique approach. They might have heard that the bonesetters here use more than just their hands, or that they call on a higher power, or even that they succeed where medicine fails. Whatever their early sense of things, they quickly learn that Tz'utujiil bonesetters have a distinct way of working, including that their diagnosis of injuries seems almost preternatural. But local bonesetters do not try to mystify anyone when they work. They simply try to treat people with the knowledge that their skills are divinely bestowed. So while it is true that many people needing care journey to San Pedro La Laguna or San Juan La Laguna because they have limited amounts of money and distrust clinicians, these are not the only reasons they make the trip, or even the main ones. By visiting the bonesetters who call Lake Atitlán home, injured people are effectively seeking out not just bodyworkers but caregivers grounded in the sacred. They are pursuing treatment from someone whose work grows from a sacred calling, something otherwise unusual in bonesetting.

This sacred approach to bonesetting stands out because, generally speaking, bonesetting practice is very empirical. It normally rests on very physical principles and practices. When a sense of the sacred does appear in a localized bonesetting tradition, then, we are reminded of how "nonsacred" most of bonesetting today actually is. This chapter explores not only how bones and bonesetting express sacrality among Tz'utujiil Mayas of San Pedro La Laguna and San Juan La Laguna but also how bonesetters from these two places have put that sacrality to practical use. In their way of thinking, their work is as much about honoring their sacred calling as it is about offering their manual care to the people who need it.

Over the years, as I was developing my interest in Maya bonesetting, I learned that many bonesetters lived and worked in San Pedro La Laguna (Paul 1976), so in 1998 I revisited the town in hopes of meeting some. Following a few leads there, I met three male bonesetters—Flavio, Victorino, and Lázaro—as well as two female bonesetters, Magda and Manuela, one of whom was the daughter of one of the male bonesetters. I tried interacting with these bonesetters as much as I could, and watched them at work when possible. Fortunately, the bonesetters liked talking about their work, so I returned to the two towns in 1999 and located two additional bonesetters, Cipriano and Martín, in San Juan La Laguna. I followed up with yearly visits to these communities, and in 2001, during a trip to San

Juan La Laguna, I was able to meet another female bonesetter, Imelda, the daughter of one of the bonesetters I had met there in 1999. The following year, 2002, I then met two additional bonesetters in San Pedro La Laguna, Raquel and Javier, the latter the son of a male bonesetter I had met four years earlier.

During my stays in San Pedro La Laguna and San Juan La Laguna, I witnessed some eight treatment encounters. These took place both in homes and in public spaces. I also saw twenty-eight other treatments performed by a San Pedro La Laguna bonesetter while he was tending to clients in Santiago Atitlán, a neighboring Tz'utujiil Maya community. Bonesetters in San Pedro La Laguna and San Juan La Laguna also described to me the interactions they had with about twenty-three specific clients. From their accounts, and from what other local people told me about treatments they had heard of or received themselves, I captured a better sense of how bonesetters work and the problems they treat. And from the bonesetters' own narratives, I quickly learned that the objects known as *baq* figure centrally in their therapeutics.

Introducing the *Baq*

Tz'utujiil Maya towns on Lake Atitlán are home to bonesetters with a sacred calling. Bonesetters there manipulate the body but always with a certain object in their hands—the *baq* or *hueso*, as first reported by Rodríguez Rouanet (1969:62). This "bone" may be an actual bone, such as a small animal vertebra, or a stone. When the bonesetter is called to treat a client, either at his or her home or out of town, he or she must bring the object along. After the client has told the bonesetter about his injury, the bonesetter will bring out the object. Depending on what part of the client's body is injured, the bonesetter will then place the baq, usually wrapped in a red cloth, on it and begin a diagnostic procedure (Hinojosa 2004c; McMahon 1994; Paul 1976; Paul and McMahon 2001). The client watches, and feels, as the object moves about his or her skin, pressing into the flesh, and changing directions. The bonesetter might point out that he or she is not moving the object; it is moving itself, receiving information directly from the suffering body. The knowledge conveyed from this object to the bonesetter's own body will then guide the bonesetter in pressing the object at points on the body where he thinks manipulation is needed.

The baq is the hallmark of San Pedro La Laguna and San Juan La Laguna bonesetting, and local people say the object makes itself known to people

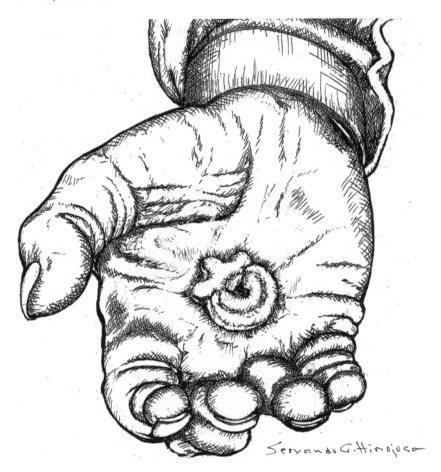

Figure 3.1. The *baq*, a revealed object used by bonesetters of San Pedro La Laguna and San Juan La Laguna. Drawing courtesy of Servando G. Hinojosa.

who are predestined to become bonesetters. How it might do this is illustrated by the testimony of Lázaro from San Pedro La Laguna. He provided this account to me in written form when I first visited his home.[1]

"ESTA ES MI HISTORIA"
Cuando naci traigo una cosa en mi mano, y cuando estoy grande me dijeron que Dios me a dado un don, y asi pasó el tiempo, de ahí empezé a soñar y una noche soñé un hombre me hablo y me dijo; que yo fuera a las doce del día a la montaña a traer una cosa y me dijo que yo no me asustara, a las doce del día me fui y cuando llegué a la montaña vi cuando salió el hueso en la

tierra salto lo recogí y regrese en la casa, ensendí una candela e insiencio y
después lo guarde. Para unos meses y empeze otra vez a soñar, soñé que un
hombre empezó a formar una calavera cuando el señor me dijo ahora le toca
usted a formar los huesos de la calavera y empeze a formar y me obligó a
que yo trabajara y empeze a trabajar.

UN DÍA MARTES 12 DE FEBRERO DE 1988

CURADOR DE HUESO: LÁZARO

[TRANSLATION] THIS IS MY ACCOUNT

There was an object in my hand when I was born, and when I grew up they
told me that God had given me a don [gift], and time went by and I began
to have dreams and one night a man appeared [in my dream] and addressed
me and told me that I should go to the mountain/forest at twelve noon to
find and bring something, telling me not to be frightened, [and] at twelve
noon I went and when I arrived at the mountain/forest I saw emerge the
hueso from the ground [and] it jumped and I collected it and returned to
my house, I lit a candle and some incense and then stored it for safekeep-
ing. Some months later I began to dream again, I dreamed that a man began
forming an entire skeleton and then he told me, "It is now up to you to
arrange the bones of the skeleton" and I began to assemble them and he
compelled me to work and so I began to work.

Tuesday, 12 February 1988

BONE CURER: Lázaro

Lázaro added that both of the baq that he now uses actually "jumped up"
from the path that day. He also explained that the *calavera* (skull) he saw
in the dream was actually an entire skeleton, standing upright like a man.
His case typifies the revelatory experience of Tz'utujiil Maya bonesetters.
The birth sign, the baq, the teacher, and the skeleton-in-the-dream recur
in the narratives of many local bonesetters. In his brief but seminal article,
Benjamin Paul (1976) reported that initiatory elements such as the latter
three leave a strong impression and feed the sense that the bonesetter
has a gift. And although Paul (1976) traced the use of the baq back to the
early twentieth century in San Pedro La Laguna, residents there and in
San Juan La Laguna seem to link the object with much older spiritual
practices tied to the sacred landscape, as Lázaro's testimony suggests. Virtually every bonesetter in the two towns uses the *sacra* (object possessing
magical potentiality). The baq may be found, or it may be inherited, but
whenever a bonesetter places it on the body, it becomes his or her vehicle
for diagnosing the injury and for treating it. Several visits to the bone-

setter may be needed for some injuries, and the bonesetter will use the baq each time.

Bonesetters from the lake area have different ways of handling the baq when diagnosing and treating clients. Some—Lázaro, Flavio, and Cipriano—will diagnose and treat using one baq. Others, for example, Victorino, might use one or two baq at the same time, depending on whether the treatment area is small (e.g., finger) or large (e.g., knee). Most baq are small enough to be carried in one's pocket, and indeed most bonesetters carry their baq wherever they go. This may be one reason that people from many towns come to learn about the Lake Atitlán–area bonesetters: even when lake-area bonesetters travel and work outside of their home towns, they take their baq with them and use it whenever they practice. The baq thus constitute a highly recognizable accoutrement of the San Pedro La Laguna and San Juan La Laguna *wikol baq*, or *curandero de hueso*.

The Baq, the Don, and Body Knowledge

It is equally telling that local bonesetters attribute a deep connection with body knowledge to the baq. It links them with the pains and structural disruptions in the client's body (Hinojosa 2004b), realities that can only be felt, and only by persons who rightfully own the sacred object they handle. A researcher in nearby Santiago Atitlán in the 1960s said that the most famous baq in San Pedro La Laguna's history may have even been a human bone (Douglas 1969:144), something that might explain how it could connect so well to the bodies it was placed on and heal them.[2] What we do know is that for many Tz'utujiil Mayas, the baq is a divine conduit for bodily knowledge and healing potential.

Some bonesetters voice this quality of the baq in revealing language. Imelda, a bonesetter and daughter of Martín, says that when she examines a client, her hand first "searches" the person's body "to see if it's broken." Then she applies the baq to the person's body. At this point, she insists, the baq or hueso itself searches out the bones within the body. "El hueso es que busca el hueso . . . [E]l hueso es como imán" (The hueso is what searches for the bone . . . [T]he hueso is like a magnet), as she puts it. The baq detects the bones within and whatever might be wrong with them. It locates them, links to them, and even pulls on them. (I will return to this attribute of the baq in chapter 4.) For her there is little question that the baq changes and repairs things when she puts it on a body. This direct application of the bone sacra partly recalls how a Yucatec Maya healer reported by Morris Steggerda and Barbara Korsch (1943:55) would rub a human tooth onto a person's ailing tooth in order to heal it. While in the Yucatec case, the healing bone had to be human, in Tz'utujiil practice what matters is that the bone be a revealed object. In the latter case, Tz'utujiils value the sacra chiefly because it can directly communicate with the body, diagnose the problem within, and change conditions inside the body. This contrasts with the tooth's potentiality in the Yucatec case. Steggerda and Korsch (1943) speak of the tooth's instrumental qualities, but make no mention of any diagnostic properties.[3]

In San Pedro La Laguna and San Juan La Laguna, that the baq goes beyond exercising the instrumental role in the Yucatec case is made clear by the way people talk about it. Although the baq is best known for effectuating a deep bodily connection between healer and sufferer, this object is also linked to a larger faculty of knowing. This faculty is suggested in narratives that express that the baq exercises a certain volition in the hands of the right person, especially in accounts detailing that the object exhibits hard-to-explain behavior. The baq is said to appear to selected people (in dreams and on paths), and it reportedly keeps returning to certain people or their households. Some narratives even describe how the baq will disapprove of how some people mishandle or neglect it, and might punish them. It can do this because it "knows" these things. According to Gabriel, an aspiring young bonesetter in San Pedro La Laguna, the baq also knows if the curer is playing around with it. "It is a sin if you play with it," he says. "It's as if the stone were also playing around." He fears that if he were to play with it, "perhaps it w[ould] get angry, if it's in the pocket it goes away from your don [gift, explained below] and you don't even feel it." The consequences of mishandling can be even more severe. Paul and McMahon (2001:259) describe a bonesetter who said that one of her children died shortly after playing with her hueso. In these ways the baq seems linked to a larger awareness, not just of the body being treated but of the person it bears a primary connection with (and his or her close family). And to hear locals tell it, this intuitive connection with the baq is possible only when the person who has received it was born with something unequivocal: the don.

When people of San Pedro La Laguna and San Juan La Laguna talk about the don, they are referring to the gift that certain people are said to be born with. This is usually a gift that predestines one to be a specialist: a bonesetter, a midwife, a sorcerer, and so on. The don might also show that someone is meant to be a shaman or even a transforming witch, as L. Paul and B. Paul (1975:708) documented. Bonesetters and bonesetters-to-be are normally said to have been born with the don, and individual bone-setters will usually talk about their don when describing how they came to find a baq. As with the baq, the don has a close bodily connection with the bonesetter, but one that is even closer and takes shape even earlier in the person's life, unbeknownst to him or her. This is because the bonesetter don first appears when the newborn's body first appears.

A San Juan La Laguna bonesetter, Cipriano, for example, was born with the don. He was holding this small bit of amniotic tissue in his hand when he first emerged, and the midwife and his father saw this. Knowing that just as it was bound to Cipriano's little body, it was also bound to his future, Cipriano's father wrapped up the don and put it away. When Cipriano was around twelve, his mother told him he had a don, but she did not say for what. By this time Cipriano's father had given him the tissue, so Cipriano also wondered what it was for. It was not until after he was thirty-two, when he started working as a bonesetter with a baq, that he knew which don he had received. He then knew the source of his ability: "Dios me ha dado ese don" (God has given me that don). This reaffirmed his sense of purpose and reminded him that he was, in a sense, physically bound to this path.

In Cipriano's case, we see how being born with the amniotically im-printed don seems to be a precursor to his finding the baq and entering the work of the bonesetter. This was also true for Lázaro, who reported in his *historia*, "There was an object in my hand when I was born," describing an event that occurred years before he found his own baq. Cipriano ex-presses the practical importance of his endowment: "Uso mi mano, y uso mi don que Dios me ha dado" (I use my hand, and I use the don that God has bestowed upon me). His hands could not physically do what they do were it not for the don that the midwife beheld the day Cipriano entered the world.

His physical connection to his gift takes yet another form. Cipriano ex-plained that his body shows certain signs. Sometimes his upper left arm twitches, and soon someone shows up needing treatment. Demonstrating a twitching arm, he explains, "Así me hace el cuerpo, y en media hora lle-gan . . . así es el seño" (My body does like this, and a half hour later they arrive . . . this is the sign). Even when he is on a trip out of town, "el seño da, el cuerpo da el seño, que así va haber algo hoy" (the sign happens, the body gives the sign, that something will happen today). For him, the don, like the baq, ties into another level of heightened consciousness about his vocation, even though it began expressing itself only after he began working.

Magda, a bonesetter from San Pedro La Laguna, who found and uses a baq, professes a different premonition about clients. She says that her dreams tell her that people are coming to see her, and they do come. But while she finds this interesting and admits that her dreams do give her pause, for most local bonesetters dreams matter for an entirely different reason. Dreams awaken them to new responsibilities, pulling back the curtain on something they have previously only walked along the edges of. They also place them on a stage where they will be put to the test.

Dreams and Validation

Practical and sacred elements work in striking concert in the validating moments that Tz'utujiil bonesetters report. As in Lázaro's case, some dream of a skeleton. Sometimes it is put together before the dreamer's eyes, or it appears in assembled form. The skeleton then collapses into a heap (Paul 1976:78). The dreamer is then instructed by someone to re-assemble the skeleton, bone by bone. The male presence in San Juan La Laguna bonesetter Martín's dream told him, "You have to rebuild it, but with this, this is a gift from God . . . this was not made by the hand of man." The presence was referring to the baq that Martín had found on a path late one night. In the dream, Martín assembled the skeleton's feet first, then worked his way up and rebuilt the skeleton and the skull. The voice then told him, "Now you know. Whoever comes to you, you must attend to them." His divine tutor's lesson was realized six months later, long after Martín had forgotten this dream, when his father-in-law told him that Martín's brother-in-law had broken his leg and needed his help.

The dreams are even more compelling when a recognizable personage appears, especially when this being can presage events and shape will. This happened to Flavio from San Pedro La Laguna, who recalled having two such dreams. In the first one a *señor* spoke to Flavio and told him he was going to find a baq in the road. The next day at noon Flavio went out to look, and sure enough, he found it. He said that the señor who appeared to him was Jesus Christ, who wore cloths and roses in the dream. The second dream was a little different. Instead of being directed to a sacred object, Flavio found himself getting chastised. Jesus Christ, who this time appeared as a very old man, told Flavio that he *had* to work, that he *had* to go out with the people to heal them. In those days, Flavio explained to me, he was resisting the call to heal. He did not want to help people. But he soon found himself becoming ill. Flavio would eat but he could not maintain his body weight, and as he grew worse he knew he had to rethink his position. It was after this second dream that he developed the will to cure and was himself cured.

After this Flavio had no more dreams with Christ, but he kept thinking about him, reflecting on how "a person has his angel, too, a caregiving angel, a guardian [angel]." Sometime after the dreams, he prayed before his altar one night and asked this angel (as he now thought of Christ) for help, asking that he engender goodwill in him. He later credited the dreams with helping him take some much-needed steps forward. Underlining the visual quality of these moments, Flavio said his dreams with Christ were really unforgettable, just like seeing a photographic image. They made a strong visual impression on him, opening him up to a role that he at first thought he could just push away.

Flavio had warm memories of his dreams, and in retrospect he knew he needed the chastising. Other bonesetters likewise remember this part of their dreams, how they were somewhat coerced into the curing role. Dreams are known to rebuke and admonish people who do not accept their calling. Like with Flavio, Martín had also been reluctant to accept his calling. Even when he became sick, he resisted. It was in this context that he received the dream about the skeleton mentioned above. He had found a baq, but he had put it away and did not want to practice with it. This is when he beheld a large man in his dream, someone he had never seen before, and this man told Martín, "You have good *suerte* [luck, fate], you have abandoned it, it has its *fortuna* [fortune, promise], you have abandoned it." Martín replied, "No," but the man said, "Yes, where have you placed it?" Martín then produced the baq, and the man continued, "This is your don, which God has given you from the womb of your mother." He then straightaway showed Martín the skeleton that he had to reassemble. After this, and after people started bringing their injuries to him, Martín resolved to help others.

Even someone with relatively little bonesetting experience, such as Gabriel, knows that bad things can happen when someone refuses his or her gift. He said of individuals gifted with the "stone" (baq) and the don, "Si no curamos la piedra se va lejos de nosotros, nos enfermamos, ya no nos curamos, nos hinchamos, tiene sueños horribles, como si yo en la cárcel y alguien allí dice, ¡¿'por qué rechasaste ese dinero?!'" (If we don't cure, the stone will go far away from us, we get sick, we can't get well, we get swollen up, we have horrible dreams, as if I were in jail and someone there says, 'Why did you reject the money?!'). Gabriel leaves little doubt that the sacred suerte behind the baq will through a dream demand an accounting from those who refuse. He adds, "It is the don of the stone."

Whereas many dreams attune curers-to-be to a future role and even compel them to carry it out, some dreams appear as variations on this theme. They might not be a definitive call to the role of bonesetter, but they reveal things that would make sense to a legitimate curer. We see this with Magda, whose dreams alerted her to future clients. Victorino, meanwhile, dreamed not about clients but about something else he was interested in. One day while I was visiting him, he reached into a pot he kept at his bedside and took out a red bundle. From the bundle he then removed two pieces of what looked like sharp-edged quartzite and what looked like a marble with a yellow swirl in it. When I said the word *canica* (marble), his granddaughter said that it was not a marble, that he had found it. He then related to me that around 1990, years after he began bonesetting, he saw his deceased parents in a dream. They had a tiny glass ball resembling a *boliche* (another word for marble), and they put it in his hand. For thirteen days, he dreamed of his parents giving him the glass object. On the thirteenth day he decided to go into the forest, where he "entered the volcano" and found the glass object. Victorino's granddaughter reiterated that though the object looks like a boliche, it is not, that these things are found in the volcano. Much to my surprise she also said that Victorino wanted to give it to me but that he could not. While he clearly did not have the same attachment to this object that he had to the baq he used for healing, the boliche was still a revealed object that came to him from the place that had yielded many other sacra. Dreams had brought it to Victorino, and even though it was not a baq, it was still bound to him. For the time being it had to stay by his bed, in the company of his other revealed objects.

Dream elements also feature prominently in Tzotzil Maya bonesetting, and bear some similarity to those of Tz'utujiil Mayas. Among Tzotzil Mayas of Larráinzar, Chiapas, for example, a person might encounter the need to urgently treat someone's bodily injury. The would-be-curer might then dream that his or her spirit travels to a sacred mountain where the ancestral gods reveal the secrets of bonesetting, or the person might recall an earlier dream in which a teacher sent by the ancestral gods instructed him or her in bonesetting (Holland 1962:238). With this validation, the person will be able to treat the injury presented. But while Tzotzil bonesetters value dreams as vehicles of learning and validation, their dreams do not reveal sacred objects to them in the way they do to Tz'utujiil bonesetters. Bonesetters in San Pedro La Laguna and San Juan La Laguna do recognize, though, that their skills are divinely bestowed and so continue to hold revelatory dreams and revealed objects in high regard. But even though the treatment of bones is predicated on something different for bonesetters in the lakeside towns than it is for Kaqchikel Maya bonesetters in Comalapa, curers from both places make use of another resource: commercial drugs.

The Use of Commercial Drugs

Even though a spiritual approach undergirds local bonesetting, bonesetters do not reject commercially available drugs. In fact, bonesetters use a sizeable array of analgesic and anti-inflammatory drugs, as well as other commercial products that are applied directly to the body. Perhaps more than any other local bonesetter, the very busy Lázaro regularly recommends and uses store-bought drugs. He especially likes Reumetan (NSAID, analgesic), which he calls a "bone pill." During his rounds and home visits in neighboring Santiago Atitlán, he would treat individuals and then sell them blister packs of ten, twenty, or thirty Reumetan capsules, almost routinely. Although he sells the drugs at a lower cost than what his clients would have to pay locally for them, it is clear that he has to invest a considerable sum of money for them up front. This suggests that Lázaro enjoys steady returns on his sales of Reumetan.

Less often, he offers another drug product to his clients. One day in Santiago Atitlán, an elderly client asked Lázaro for an injection, to which he responded that he had not brought any and that he could offer one only the following week. In lieu of an injection, she then asked him to sell her ten Reumetan capsules, which he did. After we left the woman's house, and as we were walking down the street, I asked Lázaro if he indeed gives injections. Looking a bit sheepish, he told me that he does and went on to explain that he has given clients injections of Dolo-Fenil (NSAID, analgesic, antipyretic). He applies these injections in the arm or buttocks, and not in the veins. Lázaro administers these intramuscular injections every three days for what he calls *dolor de hueso*, bone pain. He conveyed the sense that some clients really benefit from these injections.[4]

This response contrasted, however, with his reaction to this subject when I brought it up a year later. When I asked about injections, he stated flat out that he cannot and does not administer injections, making no mention of our earlier conversation. He did add, though, that his brother-in-law, who owns a pharmacy, can apply injections, as pharmacy workers are often asked to do.[5] From this changed position, I surmised that Lázaro either does not give injections anymore (and chooses to outsource them), or just does not want word to get around that he does give injections. At any rate, his administration of drugs is probably one reason he prefers not to interact with the local health center and its resident physician.

Another bonesetter who uses drugs is of a different mind when it comes to contact with physicians. Cipriano, of San Juan La Laguna, says that he asked a physician for pills to give to clients for their pain and to help them sleep. According to Cipriano, the physician told him to buy Neo-Melubrina (an analgesic, antipyretic drug), which Cipriano has since been using. This bonesetter claims that Neo-Melubrina *corta el dolor, da sueño* (relieves the pain, induces sleep). Without specifying the dose, he says that the drug should be given once an hour when the client is in pain. Cipriano knows the medication works because when he asks his clients how they are doing the day after his treatment, they say the drug is helping. Such is his clients' confidence in Cipriano's knowledge of drugs that some have asked him to give them anesthesia before he manipulates them. But he takes issue with this request because anesthesia only *hace dormir a la carne, pero al hueso no* (puts the muscle to sleep, but not the bone). A physician once told him this, Cipriano says, and he has also seen it firsthand. When he applies the baq to someone with local anesthesia, it still hurts them. He even remembers beginning to manipulate someone who was under general anesthesia (applied by a physician), only to have the person wake up screaming.[6] Needless to say, these episodes have convinced him that anesthesia is not helpful in the long run.

For the bonesetter Imelda, from San Juan La Laguna, however, anesthesia has its uses. In her view, a local anesthesia injection is warranted only when there is a lot of pain in the injured area. If the anesthesia is not used, the area will hurt a lot when she puts her hands on it. She stresses that she would not inject the anesthesia herself; someone else has to do it. For her, fortunately, most of the time this degree of pain relief is not needed. If a person is brought to her in a seriously injured state, she gives them a "prescription" to buy "bone medicine" at the pharmacy. She has them buy Dolorin (an anti-inflammatory, analgesic drug). Fifteen minutes after clients take a five-hundred-milligram tablet of this, Imelda explains, she can physically manipulate them. The drug works pretty fast, she says, and need be taken only once every twenty-four hours. It does not replace a *sobada* (massage); rather, it prepares the body *for* a sobada by offering pain relief. After she applies her massages, Imelda says that her clients can take Neo-Melubrina pills for follow-up pain. In cases of serious injury with a lot of pain, the client can take Neo-Melubrina both before and after the massage.[7]

In contrast to the commercial drugs these curers use, other more common commercial products have become mainstays in local bonesetting. Flavio, for example, likes to use hydrogen peroxide. It is second in importance only to his baq, and he describes it as "número uno" in his practice.

He eagerly finds and shows me his bottle, then describes how he uses it "to clean, to cure," to treat swelling, and even to treat fractures. He always applies it in conjunction with manual manipulation. Flavio sticks to non-invasive products such as hydrogen peroxide and some other balms and stays completely away from injections. "Those require study," he says of the latter. Like Flavio, Victorino gives primary importance to his baq but also uses commercially available products. In fact, when I encountered him on the street one day, he reached into his shirt pocket to show me the two items he never goes without: a baq and a small blue container of Balsámico GMS. When he is treating someone at home, he might also reach for the jar of Cofal he keeps on his bedside table.

In contrast, Lázaro expressly stays away from Balsámico GMS and Cofal, saying that these ointments are "very strong, very hot" and that people do not want them. He uses another product instead. One day he showed me a plastic bottle of Coppertone Sport SPF 8 sunblock cream that somebody had given him and asked me what it was for. After I explained that it was normally used for protection from sunburn, I ventured that it was probably good for lubricating the hands. He then said that this cream is good and smooth and, most important, it is not hot. It is quite cold, he stressed, adding that "the people want this." As he went on to explain its use, it became clear that he favored this product because it offered the curer a measure of protection, too. He said that when you use Cofal and then you touch cold water, the cold water will affect you. Since Cofal is a warming, hot ointment, having it on your hands when you touch cold water can invite a sudden coldness into your body. But since the Coppertone cream is already cold, then touching cold water will not harm the person who has handled it. Although he did not say it, by using the Coppertone cream on his clients, he may be trying to avoid exposing his clients to "hot" products that can make his clients vulnerable to cold later on.

The logic of using products that feel "cold" might explain why he also uses certain other commercial items. After treating a woman's shoulder one day, he applied Vicks VapoRub cream to his hands and rubbed her shoulder thoroughly with it. He showed me the small tube that it came in. And although he did not use it on this occasion, he kept a bottle of rubbing alcohol by his bed, together with adhesive medical tape and an assortment of gauzes. While these are common household products, he showed me one item that was not likely to be found elsewhere. Handing me a tube of homeopathic Calendula ointment that a gringo had given him, Lázaro said that it was really good and asked if I could bring him more. He did not say how he used it, but his use of other products suggests that he has already managed to incorporate it into his palette of tools.[8]

Bonesetters at Work

Victorino

Compared to other Maya bonesetters, Victorino got started late in life. He was almost fifty when he found a baq and did not begin practicing as a curer until a few years later. I learned this as we sat in his San Pedro La Laguna home, in the room where he slept and kept his revealed objects. As we were talking, he decided to show me what was probably the most important of these objects. He picked up a small box he kept on his altar and removed a tiny vertebra, brown and smooth from handling, for me to see. Just a centimeter and a half wide, the tiny bone had become practically an extension of Victorino himself in the approximately twenty-five years since he found it *pa juyu'* (in the hills/forest). He showed a real affinity with this baq, but the more we spoke the clearer it became that he was especially receptive to revealed objects. The Earth had yielded other objects to him, from ceramic vessels, to glass spheres, to obsidian cores, to pieces of quartzite. He said that every week he went into a cave, at a place he calls *ru chi' juyu'* (mouth of the hill). Some days the place opened to him, and other days it closed, his granddaughter added, but it is through this portal that the volcano bestowed these objects on Victorino, and he gladly stewarded them.

He did not use all of these objects in curing, but those that he did were revealed to him over a stretch of time during which his overall knowledge of bonesetting grew. One piece of knowledge he acquired over the years, and that he was especially keen to share with me, was that all the bones in the body can separate at the joint. This was particularly true of the shoulder, hip, knee, and ankle. But through experience gained, Victorino was able to leverage his knowledge about how to bring these disarticulated bones back together. He described how, when a person with a dislocation would come to him, he would take the measured steps of unwrapping the injury site, inspecting for swelling, checking the range of motion, touching with the baq, pressing around or along the injured limb, and rebinding. Then, deciding that a description was not enough, he proceeded to demonstrate this treatment on me.

Victorino took my right hand, palm down, and sandwiched it between his two hands. With one hand he supported my hand from below, while with his other hand on top he felt and pressed down on my metacarpals, trying to sense if any bones were broken or out of place. He would normally apply a cloth wrapping after this, he said. He next demonstrated how he would treat me if I had a dislocated shoulder. Taking a baq in his right hand, he partly lifted my left arm laterally, placed his hand in my left

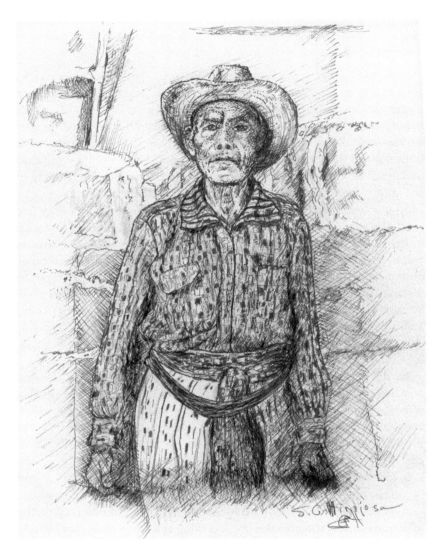

Figure 3.2. The bonesetter Victorino, of San Pedro La Laguna. Drawing courtesy of Servando G. Hinojosa.

armpit and pushed up with the baq, in a move apparently intended to lift the proximal end of the humerus. Victorino then lowered my arm, placed his hands flat against the front and back of my shoulder, and rubbed while pressing his hands together. This move, "sólo suave se hace" (has to be done gently), without traction, he said, adding that he is currently performing this treatment on a child who fell off a chair. Victorino was also known to use more than one baq at the same time. He demonstrated on himself how to sandwich the knee with two flat circular baq and push inward from the inner and outer side, rubbing each side in a circular motion.

With a broken limb, though, he needed to be more careful. To treat a broken arm, Victorino said he would first move the baq over the injury, something that made the swelling subside. He would then rub the length of the corresponding bone with Cofal. Following this, he would brace it and stabilize it with strong cardboard and wrap a bandage around it. In some fracture cases he might make the splint out of sticks that he tied together with wire. Every three days after this he would apply a light sobada to the area, for a total of fifteen days. He lamented, as other bonesetters do, that in the hospital they put casts on fractures but do not fix the broken bone. Victorino's treatment of broken fingers was also abbreviated. He would massage the fingers without traction and would wrap them for three to five days with a cloth, in a manner that he demonstrated on my hand.

Victorino showed the latter method a day or two later, when I accompanied him to a client's house. He sat down before a young man, about age twenty-five, who about a month before had been drinking and tripped and fell on a path. The middle bone of his right thumb broke, Victorino said, and had become swollen and painful. The man kept his hand wrapped up in a handkerchief and was now eager for the bonesetter to work on it and for me to watch. Victorino unwrapped the man's hand and worked the baq around the man's thumb, pressing around its perimeter. The man twisted and turned in his chair, suppressing laughter and pain while his friends goaded him. Victorino then stopped, applied Balsámico to the thumb and surrounding area, and reapplied the handkerchief wrapping. The man's friends gave him an encouraging laugh when it was over.

Back at his own house, Victorino took another opportunity to show me how he treats injuries, in this case of a young man who took a hit to his inner right knee about nine days before when playing fútbol. Victorino sat the client, about age twenty-two, down on Victorino's own bed and took out a baq. He then took the baq and applied it directly to the impact site on the inner side of the knee. When Victorino pressed the baq into the popliteal region behind the knee, the man voiced pain, but Victorino continued pressing it for a short while longer. With the pressing over, Victorino then applied Balsámico to the back and side of the knee, and wrapped a long cloth around the area. He then told the man to lie down and rest. Victorino had already treated him twice a day since the mishap; the man said that after the first few days of treatment, he was back on his feet and able to walk with a cane. He still had a limp, he said, but he was doing much better.

Victorino always looked engaged and eager to talk about his work. Even when his own body ailed him, or when alcohol got the better of him, he would put down whatever he was doing to attend to those who came looking for him. The work even seemed to help him when he was at a personal low. One day when Victorino was sick and could barely get out of bed, his granddaughter suggested that if I knew anyone who was injured, I should send them to him. She also asked if I were *golpeado* (injured by a blow) and needed his help. Whatever his changing state might be, Victorino left his door open to all comers up until his passing at seventy-four.

Lázaro

When Lázaro hands me a typed statement, I know right away he takes his credibility seriously. I have just asked him how he began as a bonesetter, when he reaches over to a table and finds the sheet of paper. The page outlines how, when Lázaro was about forty, a teacher in a dream told him that he had to go bring something from the mountain. Lázaro went to the mountain and found a "bone." Months later Lázaro began to dream of a man who assembled a skeleton and who then told Lázaro to arrange the bones as he did. Then the man told Lázaro to do this for others. Now, at fifty, Lázaro has been acting on this sublime endorsement of his path for ten years. And during those ten years some rather unexpected artifacts have come his way.

Rummaging through a drawer, Lázaro takes out some radiographic films to show me. The films, which he holds up against a sunny window, show images of serious fractures. He tells me that the man in the images was hurt in a car accident. The victim got the images taken and then came to Lázaro, who says that he "fixed" the man. But before going into details, Lázaro shows me the object he uses to fix people with. He reaches into his pocket and removes one of the baq that he uses and places it in my hand. Looking at the bone closely, I can make out its flattened sides, overall squarish shape, and brown patina. Lázaro says that it comes from a knee. He then produces another baq that is wrapped up in a red cloth, but does not place it in my hand. As I later come to see, this concealed baq

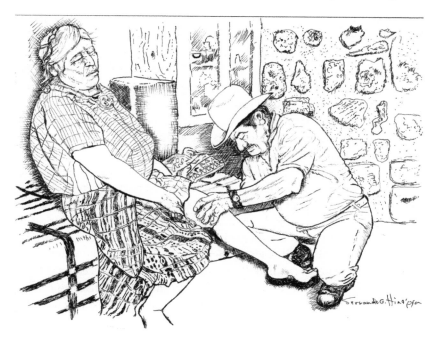

Figure 3.3. The bonesetter Lázaro, of San Pedro La Laguna, treating an elderly client's knee. Drawing courtesy of Servando G. Hinojosa.

delivers the bulk of his diagnostic and treatment activity, and he keeps it close for this reason.

Over the course of different field seasons by the lake, I see more treatments performed by Lázaro than by any other area bonesetter. This is partly because of his friendly disposition but more because of the sheer volume of clients he works with. He deals with injuries virtually every day, making him feel proficient enough to say that while fractures are difficult to cure, dislocations are relatively easy to treat. The forms these injuries come in have also alerted him to revealing bodily signs that help with diagnosis and treatment. Besides noting the deformity an injury can cause, and how the client reports pain, for instance, he has learned to listen to the body directly. When he treats a person with a painful shoulder, he can feel and hear the manner in which "truena el hueso" (the bone clicks). This crepitus immediately tells him there is a structural problem in this joint. Lázaro also looks out for swelling, since this means that he needs to apply heat to the area.[9] He has also learned that to effectively treat a leg injury, during the treatment he must get the person to move his or her toes.

I see the attention he pays to the details of individual cases during visits to neighboring Santiago Atitlán. Taking a boat from one of San Pedro La Laguna's docks, Lázaro goes to Atitlán every Tuesday and Friday to see clients. I accompany him a few times and notice how people are usually waiting for him at the Atitlán dock, ready to take him to their house. People also call out to him as he is walking down the street, so he winds up making many unscheduled visits to homes. During one such home visit he gives a follow-up treatment to someone who broke his clavicle a month earlier. The client, an older teen who got injured while playing, now sits while Lázaro applies his third treatment to him.

Lázaro first unwraps the ACE bandage binding the young man's shoulder, uncovering a small bit of paper padding taped to the broken left clavicle. Some cloth padding is also removed from the armpit of the affected shoulder. Lázaro then rerolls the bandage he removed and puts it aside; next he removes the padding taped to the fracture site. Reaching into his pocket, Lázaro extracts his cloth-covered baq, kisses it, and places it on the clavicle. He holds the baq directly on the fracture site, leaves it there for a few seconds, and then begins pushing the baq against the clavicle from the front. Lázaro asks the client if it is hurting. The young man grimaces but says no. Lázaro then places his left hand on the clavicle and presses the baq against the base of the man's neck. Moving the baq to his left hand, the bonesetter then holds the baq against the clavicle and slowly lifts up the client's left arm laterally. He then slowly lowers the arm, all the while checking to see that the fracture union site does not move. Seeing it is stable, Lázaro feels the alignment of the fracture with his hand, then reapplies the baq to the fracture site. By this time the client has been lowering his head, so Lázaro asks him to straighten up. He presses the baq to the clavicle once more and then applies Coppertone cream, but only to the skin along the length of the collarbone. Once the manipulation is complete, Lázaro takes a section of toilet paper from a roll he keeps in his shoulder bag and folds it into a tight square pad, one and half inches each side. He then places this square pad atop the upper surface of the fracture site, takes some masking tape from his bag, and secures it to the shoulder. Lázaro follows up with more tape, adhering it to skin areas devoid of any cream. Once the pad is taped down, he rewraps the ACE bandage over the man's shoulder, across the chest, and under the arms, clipping it behind his back. With assurance that Lázaro will return in a few days, he and I take our leave.

During another trip to Atitlán Lázaro brings me to a client whose treatment is largely completed and whose injuries were far more serious. At a music-cassette stall in the town market we meet a man in his twenties, originally from Chichicastenango, who three years before had been in a terrible accident. Riding his bicycle, he was struck by a moving truck. The impact fractured both bones of his lower right leg, lacerated the knee, and broke both of his left forearm bones at midshaft. By his telling, he was taken to the National Hospital in Sololá, where they took X-rays of the injuries and stitched his knee. The physicians also placed a cast on his left arm and on his entire right leg. But when they told him that much of his right leg would have to be amputated, he knew he could not stay there. He came to San Pedro La Laguna.

When he arrived at Lázaro's house, Lázaro removed the casts and began the lengthy process of treating him. For months, Lázaro applied the baq, his hands, and Coppertone cream to the man's broken body. Alternately immobilizing and massaging the broken limbs, his hands eventually got results. Now standing in his vending stall, the man holds out his left arm for me to see, straightening it as much as possible. Only a slight bump on the forearm is visible. He then eagerly removes his boot from his right foot, rolls up his jeans, and lifts up his lower leg. A large scar and protrusion mark where the impact broke his tibia and fibula. Lázaro finds a small stool to sit on while he passes the baq over the lower leg. He applies Coppertone cream to the shin area and stands back up. These days the man says that he feels some pain, but seems more than happy to have two feet to stand on.

Lázaro sometimes shows X-ray films of this man's original injuries to those who come seeking help in his home. One field season, when I brought a student to meet Lázaro, he likewise showed her the X-rays he had first shown me. He then brought out some photos I had taken of the man he had treated to show my student how straight his arm and leg looked after treatment. The photos I was asked to take, it seems, have become part of Lázaro's legitimization before visitors.

But it is during treatment encounters that he best shows his abilities, and over the years he has enhanced these abilities by using household objects. He routinely wraps injuries with toilet paper, masking tape, cloth, towels, or whatever materials are handy. He even wraps toilet paper around pieces of wood so that it can better support the bones it is placed against. When applying an initial treatment to another older teen with a broken clavicle in Atitlán, Lázaro knows that he will have to place firm supports around the fracture site. He asks for *tablillas* (little boards), and when household members bring him one, he cuts it in half and wraps the pieces together with toilet paper. He then puts the one-and-a-half-inch-long bundle of wood atop the aligned fracture site. Lázaro then binds a

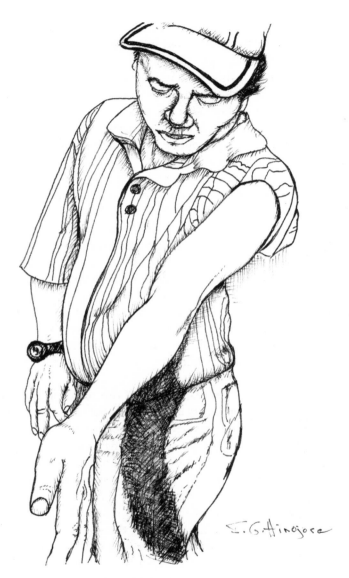

Figure 3.4. Client of Lázaro's in Santiago Atitlán showing his posttreatment fractured arm. Drawing courtesy of Servando G. Hinojosa.

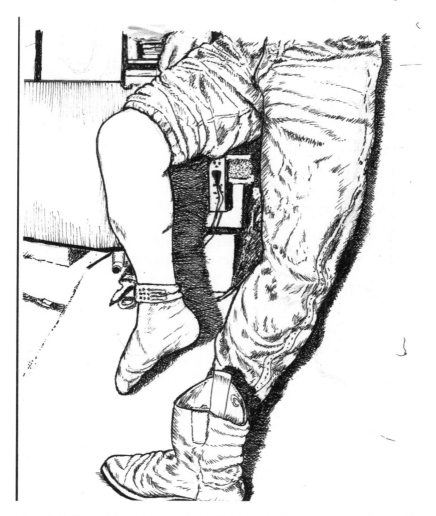

Figure 3.5. Client of Lázaro's in Santiago Atitlán showing his posttreatment fractured leg. Drawing courtesy of Servando G. Hinojosa.

cloth bandage around the client's shoulder and chest such that it pushes down on the tablilla, keeping the broken ends of the clavicle in place. The client is able to start lifting his arm a few days later.

He builds on this approach when he treats yet another older teen with a broken clavicle. After wrapping a small wooden square with toilet paper, he tapes the paper so it will not unravel. He then makes a thick square of toilet paper to use with the tablilla. Lázaro places the tablilla and the paper square on a strip of masking tape to apply to the break site. But before he does, he touches the clavicle and decides he will need to put additional support there. He folds another length of toilet paper into a roll and places it against the upper side of the fracture. Over this rolled pad he affixes the covered wooden square and the paper square, fastening them down with masking tape. After placing more tape across the stabilizing padding, he pushes down on the taped wooden square on the break to check the union site's stability. At this point the family looks for a padding to put under the sufferer's affected arm and gives Lázaro two folded white towels to place in the armpit. With the wooden square and paper and cloth padding in place, Lázaro binds the fixation pad to the clavicle with a strip of green cloth (actually a woman's belt) and wraps it over the client's shoulder, across his chest, and back over his shoulder, where he ties it.

Although Lázaro has a lot of practice at reducing clavicle fractures, he also sees many other kinds of injuries and has even found seemingly novel ways of dealing with them. For example, when he first treats the injured left forearm of a woman in her late teens, he applies the baq along the length of her forearm, really pressing it between the ulna and radius. He applies the Coppertone cream and then produces two small wooden hexagrams, which he wraps in toilet paper. After wrapping the upper forearm with toilet paper and securing it with masking tape, he then probes to find where the arm hurts the most. At this spot he tapes down one of the wrapped hexagrams, and on the exact opposite (inner) side of the forearm he applies the other hexagram. He does this, interestingly, in a manner reminiscent of the way in which separator pads are used in Chinese bonesetting (Fang et al. 1996; Shang et al. 1987). Lázaro then further affixes the wooden pieces to the forearm by wrapping a long bandage around it. To be clear, although actual separator pads are used to keep a stable space between the two long bones (radius and ulna) of the forearm when they are immobilized, the nonorthodox placement of Lázaro's hexagons does not suggest this purpose.

It is indicative, nonetheless, of an understanding of the forearm's skeletal anatomy. We see this also when Lázaro is treating a young man's injured hand. After he feels and massages the hand, Lázaro finishes by putting a paper pad between the metacarpals of the man's index and middle fingers on the dorsal side of the hand, then wrapping the hand with an elastic bandage. While there is nothing to suggest that Lázaro is separating these bones as part of the treatment, these practices pay witness to a form of experimentation with techniques, perhaps developing into a personal signature.

Lázaro feels strongly that his techniques work, so when his clients dismiss him or avoid him, he does not take it well. During one of our visits to Atitlán we go by one house expecting to see a client Lázaro had treated for a fracture. But when someone else answers the door, the person says that the client is not home. Since Lázaro had said earlier he would be coming by, though, this leaves him with a bad feeling. In fact, it really bothers him. As we walk away he grumbles that some people are *malagradecidos* (ungrateful), while others are *agradecidos* (grateful). The people at the house probably just do not want to give him an *agradecimiento* (appreciation, token payment), he says, so they pretend his client is not home. It might also be the case that the family has decided to see another bonesetter, a prospect that can unsettle Lázaro even more.

But Lázaro is familiar with this tension between bonesetters and clients, and even among bonesetters. In fact, he has participated in it. Like I reported at the start of this book, at one point Lázaro was in the process of treating a middle-aged man in Atitlán who had fallen off a truck and injured his left hip and left arm. Then a complication arose. One of the man's sons, who had been keeping watch at the window, said someone was coming. They quickly turned off the lights and told everyone to duck. The visitor appeared as a silhouette at the door, knocked for a couple of minutes, and then left. With the coast clear, Lázaro resumed his work. I later learned that the person who knocked was in fact another bonesetter (from San Juan La Laguna) who had earlier applied four treatments to the man, apparently with unsatisfying results. The family did not want her services anymore, but instead of telling her directly, they enlisted another bonesetter's help and simply pretended they were not home. The episode no doubt made the other bonesetter bristle.

This passive "firing" of a bonesetter is something bonesetters in different towns surely experience at some point or other. These dismissals give injured people a chance to try someone new, but they also harden feelings among bonesetters. For the most part, though, Lázaro is too busy working to stew over these situations. He is on the road most days of the week, making rounds in Sololá, Santiago Atitlán, San Antonio Palopó, and Tecpán. He even keeps an "office", he says, in the latter town. For now he has managed to tend to his coffee plantings when he is home on Sundays, but no matter what day of the week the boat brings him home, he will probably find someone waiting patiently at his door.

Flavio

For someone who was eager to talk about his baq, Flavio was in no hurry to show it to me. In fact, he never did. On the occasions that he described his *huesito*, though, he said it was shaped like the closed *flor de palma* flower on his altar — long, cylindrical, and tapering to a point — or that it resembled a citrus blossom. He found it on a road after a dream told him it would be there. Flavio was about thirty at the time, and that moment launched him into the work of a bonesetter for the next forty-five years. So by the time I first sat with him, when he was seventy-seven, he had had ample time to reflect on the many ways people get injured and the courses of action they should and should not take. The way he saw it, there were many people who suffered fractures and other injuries due to truck and bus accidents, and some of these were quite serious. But Flavio said that if a person with, say, a fractured leg went to a physician, the physician would just say, *vamos a cortar* (we're going to amputate). Just as problematic for him was how physicians would routinely put people in hard casts, even if their fractures were not treated first. He recalled how people came to him wearing casts, people who still needed treatment. Of such cases, he said, he "lo quité el yeso" (removed the cast) so that he could treat them himself.

As Flavio told me about some of the treatments he had performed, I commented that he must have a lot of *fuerza* (strength), in his hands. But he immediately corrected me. "No tiene fuerza que ver . . . solo suave vamos a hacer" (It doesn't have anything to do with strength . . . we just do it gently), he said with a rubbing motion of his hands. He then told me more about how he applies this measured strength in cases of injury. To treat a leg fracture, for instance, he first works the baq over the leg in a way he described as "suave un poco, no es duro" (a little gently, it isn't hard). After next applying hydrogen peroxide to the limb, Flavio would perform a relatively firm sobada, then place five-inch-long sticks along the break, which he would then bind to the leg with a cloth. The second time he would handle the fractured limb, he would do a more "normal" sobada, and by the time he would perform the third and fourth massages, the injury would already be *componiéndo(se)* (mending). His overall approach, then, was to unwrap and manipulate the injured area every three or four days, understanding that it should stay bandaged for twenty days in toto. He had seen fractures happen to many people who fell in the hills. It also happened to people involved in car accidents, as with a university graduate from Guatemala City who came to Flavio for treatment following a collision.

Flavio dealt with other injuries as people brought them to him. He re-

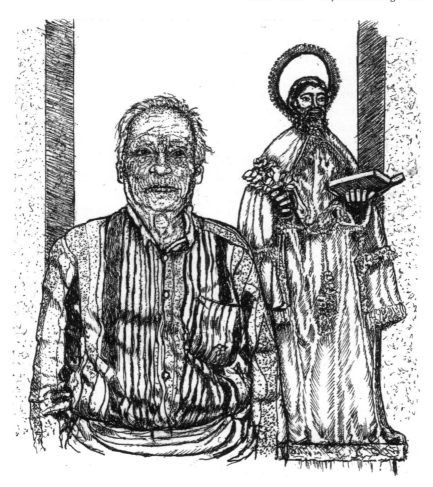

Figure 3.6. The bonesetter Flavio, of San Pedro La Laguna. Drawing courtesy of Servando G. Hinojosa.

membered that a man once came to him from the coast with an injured knee that was so swollen he could not walk. Flavio applied the baq and his hands to the knee and wrapped it. In these cases, he said, the knee should stay wrapped up for eight days. This client, it turned out, did not return after the first treatment. He probably just got better, Flavio reasoned. An injured ankle can also interfere with walking, but when it is very *nisipojik* (swollen up), it can be hard to treat. This is because when it is swollen, there is no easy place to tie a bandage or cloth around it. Flavio would still try to massage it, though, because if he did not, the sufferer would probably remain unable to walk or work, putting his or her household income at risk. Many people sprain their ankles by slipping on a trail or by losing their footing around their house, but when it is a breadwinner who falls, his or her whole family really feels the effects of the injury. Flavio's emphasis here on lower body injuries not only speaks to the reality of tricky walking surfaces but also signals how bonesetters such as himself generally take care to get people back on their feet and back to work as soon as possible.[10]

Flavio took measured steps to deal with injuries, but he also relied on a couple of natural products. When I asked him if there were *remedios* (medicines) for fractures and other impact injuries, he reached into his bag and took out a small white jar the size of a *pomada* container. It was labeled, *Crema de cascabel* (rattlesnake cream). Flavio said this cream was good for people with *golpes* (blows) and that it was even helpful for people who did not have golpes. Demonstrating a limp, he then told me how helpful it is for people that limp. But the most important natural product for him is the beef bone *manteca* (lard) he uses to work the body. Also calling it "líquido del hueso del ganado" (beef marrow liquid), Flavio stressed how invaluable it was. He showed me lump of it in a cloth, then explained that he first applies it to his hands, then heats his hands, and then applies his hands to the injury, rubbing it onto his wrist as he spoke. "Bonita para quebradura, (es) pura manteca" (It's lovely for fractures, it's pure lard), he said almost gleefully. Something about its origin also fascinated him, stressing as he did that "tiene una bendición el ganado" (cattle have a certain blessing); the blessing made the marrow product highly effective. So even though he would buy this substance at a pharmacy, he did not associate it with the world of commercial pharmaceuticals. In fact, he claimed that the marrow product was good because the grass the cattle ate was of high quality. And since they ate good grass, this made the beef very healthful. He did not appreciate, then, how physicians supposedly sold the same grass in commercial pills.

For Flavio, this was yet another example of the way physicians were motivated more by profit than by anything else. He, on the other hand, accepted what people gave him, "por voluntad nada más" (simply according to their will). His guiding outlook dictated that he not ask for payment from people because, as he put it, "la bendición de Dios es más bueno" (God's blessing is better). It would be a sin, he insisted, to ask money of those people who came to him from neighboring towns, or who asked him to go see them. Even if treating others entailed hardships of time and effort, he resolutely saw this as part of a bonesetter's duties, especially since the healing came from a sacred source. He said of the baq, "El don no quiere pisto, es pecado. Tiene un milagro el señor Jesucristo" (The gift [of the baq] isn't about money, it doesn't need money; that's a sin. It is imbued with a miracle from the Lord Jesus Christ). There was no room for profiteering in Flavio's view.

Tending to the people who came to him kept Flavio busy, as did making boat trips to Santiago Atitlán. He would travel to the neighboring town every three days or so because he wanted to treat each of his clients there four times—enough, he thought, for them to get well. Up until his later years he even found time to devote to San Pedro La Laguna's home *cofradía*. He was not the head *cofrade* at the time, but he visited with the fifteen-member group whenever he could. The work and the strain took a gradually heavier toll on him. On one occasion he told me he had been rowing and asked me if I had a remedy for his aches and pains. A year later he again told me his body was hurting. He bore the burden and duty of his don for another year and was laid to rest at around age eighty-two.

Martín

Walking around San Juan La Laguna, I found that nearly everyone knew Martín the bonesetter. For one thing, Martín had eight children and many grandchildren, which put him in many places at once, in a way. But more important, he had been setting bones for some fifty years and had no doubt treated many of the people I met in the street. With their help I eventually found his house, and I finally sat down with him in his patio. But when I asked the eighty-three-year-old how he got started, he leaned back, groaned a little, and said it was a somewhat long story. He then gave me a thorough account of the events that set him on the road to becoming a *wikol baq*.

Early one morning, he was walking to the town of Santa Clara. The sun was not up yet, so he took care to place his feet securely on the stepped path, bearing the weight of a *cacaxtle* (tumpline load) as he moved through the darkness. That is when, in his words, "I saw something like a star" in the broken road. The object seemed to jump like an animal, making him wonder what it could be. He touched it with his staff, and it went out; this made him think that it had to be an animal. Strangely, at that moment he could not even feel the weight of the load borne across his forehead. He then wiggled the object with the point of his staff, and because there was a moon out, he said, "I saw something like a white stone." As he got a better look at it, he thought, "Una cristalina que es poderosa, es buenos regalos,

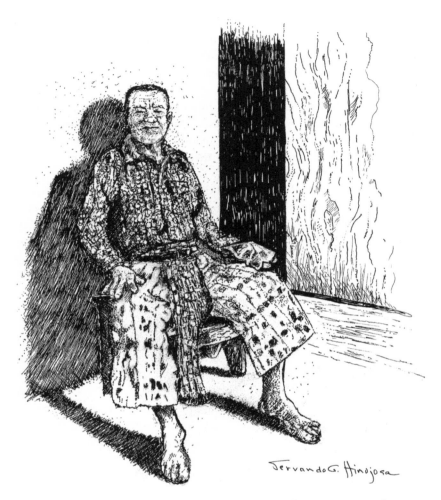

Figure 3.7. The bonesetter Martín, of San Juan La Laguna. Drawing courtesy of Servando G. Hinojosa

antes dice" (A crystalline stone which is powerful is a good gift, they used to say). So he picked up the object and placed it in his belt, and continued on his way to town. He was pleased that a man he encountered on the road shortly after this wanted to buy some of the tomatoes he was carrying.

As Martín made his way toward Santa Clara, every once in a while he would touch the stone, again thinking that it might just be an animal. When he returned to San Juan La Laguna later that day and told his mother what he had found, she commented that "hay fortuna buena, hay fortuna mala" (there are good outcomes, there are bad outcomes), where such a crystalline stone is found. She was not sure what to make of it, so she told him to put it in the house rafters. Then things took a turn for the worse. Martín became ill. For two months, he said, he did not eat. His male burro died, followed by his female burro nine days later. People thought Martín was going to die next. And because his wife, moreover, was suffering from obesity, the whole of his household felt afflicted. It was then, in the midst of this suffering, that Martín had an important dream in which a divine tutor told Martín that he had abandoned something that was actually the baq. When Martín produced the baq he had found in the road, the tutor then told Martín to behold a complete skeleton, then to reassemble it once it had collapsed, as I explained earlier. In Martín's later recollection, this all happened because he had been resisting the calling to become a healer.

This experience intensified Martín's subsequent thinking about bonesetting. More so than any other bonesetter of the area, he stressed that his work came from God, and he liked to repeat, "Yo soy servidor de Tata Dios" (I am the servant of God the Father). He was also the only lakeside bonesetter to tell me that when he cured he lit candles and burned incense, "since they are things of God." This attribution of healing power to God carried over into his encounters. At one point, he said, when he would go to heal someone, he would first pass his hand over the person's injury and commend the work to God. "I ask for the hand of God," he said of these moments.

Many people had sought him out over the years, including people from other places. He described some of the clients he had treated and took care to mention clients on the higher end of the income scale. These included a mayor of San Pedro La Laguna, and an army general who, Martín said, flew him to Guatemala City. Martín also described the time he received a formal summons from the governor of Sololá. The governor said that Martín had treated a brother of his and that a friend of the governor, a physician, now needed help. The governor sent Martín in his car to the doctor's house. There Martín treated the physician, who had impacted his tailbone when he slipped stepping out of his car. On another occasion, when Martín went to treat someone in Guatemala City, so strong an impression did he leave on a physician there that the physician reportedly wanted to buy Martín's baq, calling it a *prodigio* (a "miraculous thing"). Martín had to refuse, though, because it was a don from Tata Dios.

These were but a few instances in which the people Martín treated acknowledged his skill in some way. Each time he described a treatment, he underlined how the clients recognized his abilities and accorded him respect. It was probably important for him to tell me these validating accounts since I did not see him treat anyone. His choice to talk about people who were professionals and, moreover, from out of town was probably meant to add an extra layer of validation.

At any rate, the people he described trusted him because he apparently delivered results, and he credited his good results in part to the materials he used. But unlike other local bonesetters, Martín did not use store-bought analgesics and anti-inflammatory drugs. The only thing he bought in the pharmacy was pomada. This topical product suited him when he needed to handle limbs and perform deep-tissue massage, but it was only the most recent product that he used for this. Martín remembered that some fifty to sixty years ago, well before there were any pharmacies, he would get *tuétano de toros* (bull bone marrow) from the butcher. After cooking it and letting it cool, it would make a really good pomada. This is one area in which he has influenced his daughter Imelda, who is becoming a bonesetter in her own right. She uses the same product, calling it *líquido de res* or *grasa de toro* and notes that it works like a *pomada natural*.[11] Imelda buys this product from the butcher and says that when an injured person comes to her, she rubs it directly onto the injury. She might even apply the pomada natural to a leaf and then place the leaf on the injury. In either case, she then heats a cloth and binds it to the injury site. Most bone-setters see the benefit of warming injured limbs, and Imelda is no exception.[12] She reasons, further, that if the client's bones are dislocated, they are perforce cold, making it necessary to heat them up.

Martín imparted what he could to his daughter Imelda, and she learned a lot by watching him and by curing alongside her husband, who died eight months before I met her. Martín thus generally approved of the way she worked. This stood in contrast, though, to how he viewed other bone-setters. For the most part, he distrusted them. And while it is not unusual to hear a bonesetter voice distrust about other bonesetters, the degree to which Martín expressed suspicion about them as well as about other people in general was a bit unexpected. Referring to his own work, for example, he was emphatic about how there was always envy out there. He told me, "Siempre hay envidia, siempre hay envidia. Si uno trabaja, si uno tiene ciencia, si uno medio habla, hay envidia" (There is always envy, there is always envy. If one works, if one has exacting skill/knowledge, if one says even a little, there is envy).

He proceeded to tell me that during one feast of San Pablo, he fell into a *barranco* (gorge), just outside of town. This happened because of envidia, he insisted, adding that there is still a lot of envy out there and it is not good. But he kept a certain saying in mind: "No hay cosas que no se paga . . . hay autoridad, allí está con Dios" (Nothing escapes payback. . . . God holds final authority). It reminded him that in the end, God dispenses justice to all. This expression provided him with little consolation, though, when another misfortune befell him around 1993. Martín showed me his lower right shin, which showed signs of deformity resulting from incomplete fracture reduction. He said, without naming anyone, that certain people did this to him. One of his grandsons then said that someone had struck Martín with a machete and that the X-ray showed that it had sliced clean through his bones. The young man pointed to a cut stick to underline his point. When the attack happened, he continued, there was a lot of blood and people thought Martín was going to die. Martín said that he had to spend nine months in the hospital in Sololá, long enough for the staff there to joke that he now owned the hospital. They had to put nails in his leg, he said, showing me four circular scars. He also detailed how the medical staff put something inside his bone, describing what sounded like an intramedullary rod, to stabilize the tibia. The grandson added that they needed to operate on Martín to "remove" the object but that Martín was afraid of getting an operation.

This assault and the envy that triggered it were one of Martín's big disappointments in life, I sensed. But he tempered whatever disenchantment he knew with a certain optimism and sanguinity. He certainly conveyed this about bonesetting when he told me, "My eyes have failed me, but my hands do well." Also bearing heavily on his mind was a premonition he had about his life. God once told him in a dream, "Have patience. You have to live ten more years." When Martín first told me this in 1999, seven years had elapsed since he had had the dream. A couple of years later, he reminded me about the dream and said it had happened nine years before. He was wary that he might not be around the following year and mused on the temporality of life: "Somos puro abona, el Santo Mundo. Él nos da a uno, y vamos a Él" (We're just fertilizer [in the end], [before] the Holy Earth. He gives to one, and we go to Him). In 2002, he was happy to still be around, and he believed that part of the reason was that he did not treat bonesetting like a business. "It isn't a business," he told me. "Por eso Tata Dios me ha dado mi permiso, de quedar aquí en la tierra. Si hago de mi voluntad, no hago nada" (God the Father has allowed me to remain here on Earth for this reason. If I work because of my will alone, it amounts to nothing). He lived beyond his demise foreseen, leaving the earth at nearly ninety years of age.

The *Baq* and Generational Transmission

People from San Pedro La Laguna and San Juan La Laguna continue seeking bonesetters because of an abiding confidence they have in their hands, in their sacred tools, and in them. Knowing that these curers have deep family ties to bonesetting bolsters this confidence. When I asked the founder of San Juan La Laguna's local library, whose own grandfather was a wikol baq, about whether bonesetters tend to run in families, he nodded and said, "Se va repitiendo" (We see this again and again). This sentiment is common in the area and appears in Paul's (1976) early report about bonesetting in San Pedro La Laguna. He described a very accomplished bonesetter named Ventura. This man had experienced a series of dreams, had found a hueso, had received instructions in its use by yet other dreams, had then experienced misfortunes, and ultimately became a respected curer. When Ventura died, his hueso disappeared and ostensibly wound up in the hands of another person, a curer in San Juan La Laguna who reportedly charged high fees for his services. But because the hueso took offense at this, it took leave of this man. It then appeared in a dream to Ventura's daughter, Rosario. It told her that she was to become a bonesetter but that she should never charge her clients. Before long the bone appeared in her home, in the same spot where her father used to keep it. Following some hesitations and episodes of sickness, she became a bonesetter herself, effectively succeeding her father.[13]

Some people reference this story about Ventura when addressing how bonesetting can get transmitted across generations. But this idea also gains traction when people see transmission occurring among members of a family today. Victorino's is one such family. One day, when I was talking with Victorino about his baq, his daughter Magda said that she, too, had found a baq. She then pulled an object wrapped in red cloth out of her brassiere and showed it to me. Magda described how she found the object around 1997 and had been using it ever since. She seemed interested, in fact, not only in talking about her baq but in showing me what she had learned since she found it. When Victorino was demonstrating on me how he treats a dislocated shoulder by sticking the baq into the client's armpit and pushing up on the proximal end of the humerus, Magda stepped in and showed me her technique. She put my left arm on her right shoulder and rubbed my shoulder with both her hands, as if she were applying Cofal.

This show of enthusiasm notwithstanding, Magda and other individuals who are learning by watching a parent do not necessarily set up a separate bonesetting practice with clients right away. Rather, I got the sense that she was waiting for something to happen, biding her time. During another visit to see Victorino I asked Magda if she were still receiving people to treat. Although at first she said no, she then said that she only treats kids, not adults. Magda added that she does not do the work, or the whole extent of it, because she still has her father, Victorino. When he dies, she said, *then* she will do the work. She saw him as the pillar of bonesetting authority in the family, looming large into his final years. After Victorino died, I again spoke with Magda and learned that her curing workload had increased dramatically. I asked her if she had had any dreams about her bonesetting work. She confirmed that she had, but the dreams she described were not the kind I had come to expect. She said she dreams that people are coming to see her, and they indeed come shortly afterward.[14]

Another of Victorino's children, his son Javier, also began working in bonesetting toward the end of Victorino's life. Javier described how Victorino gave him three baq around six months before he died, and this enabled him to begin curing. Javier underlined how important the baq were for his start: "A mi me recibí porque fueron regalo de mi papá" (I entered the work because they [the baq] were a gift from my father). But the baq alone did not prepare him for bonesetting. By the time Javier received the baq, he had had ample chance to observe Victorino at work. And the learning from Victorino continued even after Victorino died. Javier recounted that "como dos o tres días después se muriera soñé también trabajando con él" (Around two or three days after he died I also dreamed that I was working with him). "He was telling me this and that" about setting bones, Javier said about his father. For him the dreams were a fitting continuation of how his father had shared so much with him, "porque aquel siempre me enseña todo" (because he was always showing me everything).

This instruction from his deceased father seemed right to Javier because, as he put it, "cuando se muere sus papás, sus mamás, siempre le ofrecen su trabajo, así, de confianza" (when someone's father, mother, dies, they always entrust their work to them [the children]). He was glad to be walking in his father's footsteps, using his father's baq. He told me of this conferral, "Estoy contento cuando me regaló. Unos tienen miedo de recibir esos huesos, y tienen miedo de curar . . . pero nosotros no tenemos miedo para nada" (I was so happy when he gave them to me. Some people are afraid to receive those *huesos*, and they're afraid to cure . . . but we're not the least bit afraid). Whereas others might be afraid to take up the work, he and his sister were not, he insisted. And his new role is working out well for him. Javier stated that in the year since his father died, he has treated around five people, including a man who could not walk but who is now working. These cases prompt him to say of his treatments that "casi ya están dando resultado" (they already seem to be producing results). Like his father, Javier even takes the baq with him whenever he travels to Guatemala City because, he says, "you never know." During our last visit he encouraged me to visit him and his sister Magda again whenever I could. Javier especially wanted me, whom he called "a friend of my father," to see him treating clients at his house.

Like we see with Magda and Javier, the children of bonesetters are ideally bold enough to take on the work, but this is not always the case. Sometimes, out of fear, they do not accept or receive the baq. Lázaro thus comments that one of his daughters in Guatemala City has a don, "pero no quiere trabajar, no se anima . . . porque curación de hueso cuesta" (but she doesn't want to work, she doesn't get interested . . . because curing bones is hard). He sounds a bit disappointed about this. Still, if his treatment encounters in Santiago Atitlán tell us anything, Lázaro is nevertheless leaving strong impressions about bonesetting on other young people. Some of those who watch him treating their family members might eventually feel drawn to the work. It is also true that to the degree that the children of bonesetters may accept the work, the acceptance may have many conditions and even be subject to modern interpretation. Cipriano's son, Roberto, for example, says that his bonesetter father has shown him how to "*agarrar*" (grab/manipulate) a little bit. But Roberto thinks that the don for curing has to come from the inside; it cannot simply be taught. He still likes the work somewhat, though. Does Roberto ever see himself becoming a bonesetter like his father? He says only that he would prefer to become a physiotherapist.

Although Cipriano's son might not become a wikol baq, whatever interest he does have likely stems from observing his father at work a lot. There is little question that observation remains an important portal of learning. I am reminded of this when Magda demonstrates a shoulder treatment on me, and I notice her young daughter Delfina watching her closely. Delfina is growing up around bonesetting and notices not only how her mother treats injuries but also how her mother always carries her baq with her, even to the market, so she can be ready to treat others should the need arise. Today, then, just as there is little doubt that Magda learned by observing her father, Victorino, it now it seems that her own daughter is learning by watching her.

Another young person in San Pedro La Laguna is also doing a lot of observing, but with the explicit aim of learning more about bonesetting.

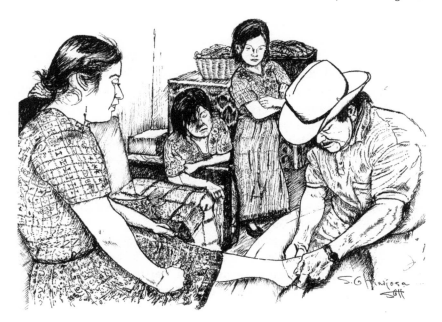

Figure 3.8. Lázaro treating a woman's foot in Santiago Atitlán. In this artistic rendering, other members of the family look on, in a manner suggestive of how people first witness Maya bonesetting techniques and later remember them. Drawing courtesy of Servando G. Hinojosa.

Gabriel thus observes his bonesetter sister, Manuela, when she treats, and he sometimes even steps in to help her out. He might help steady the client or hold his or her limb while Manuela manipulates it. All the while, he is watching, learning more. He feels he should do this because, even though he was not born with a don like his sister was, he has already found his hueso, after he fell near it. Manuela, meanwhile, is happy to help Gabriel learn, but she also tells him that he needs to practice more, that he needs to go out too, and treat other people himself.

Gabriel is an example of a person deliberately learning about bonesetting, and from a young age. His direct mode of learning might even lend support to the idea that bonesetters have been open in the past to teaching other bonesetters. But while this transmission, involving teaching and even gifting of baq to a successor, does happen, I have seen only tentative examples of this and only within families. At any rate, this mode of transmission goes against another narrative stream, which argues that when a bonesetter dies, his baq and his work leave the scene along with him (see Rodríguez Rouanet 1969:62). Raquel, from San Pedro La Laguna, for example, says that when a bonesetter dies, he takes his work with him or her (even though she knows of cases in which the bonesetter's children take up the work). Another woman, however, described an incident that suggested a more lasting tie between the bonesetter's baq and his immediate family. A woman from San Pedro La Laguna said that a bus containing *pedranos* (inhabitants of San Pedro La Laguna) and *juaneros* (inhabitants of San Juan La Laguna) once had an accident over at the highway junction, Los Encuentros. Nearly twenty people died. She then said that one of the passengers who died was a bonesetter named Pedro, who was traveling to Guatemala City to treat someone. According to Pedro's wife, Pedro had taken his baq with him that day. However, after the crash, when his wife opened the place at home where he usually kept the baq, there it was, as though it had returned home.

The bond between the baq and the bonesetter's home may be strong precisely because it grows from another, more visceral bond, one between the bonesetter and his or her parent. When Martín dreamed of a divine teacher, the teacher accordingly said of the baq Martín had found, "Esto es un tu don que te ha dado Dios desde el vientre de su madre" (This is your don which God has given you through the womb of your mother). The teacher forcefully reminded Martín that the baq manifested itself to him because he had received the don through his progenitor, his mother's womb. In his case, even though he was not born with a physical don in his hand, the don nonetheless comes from the mother. It is transmitted through her and is as such a lifelong, physically grounded gift. Martín was thus born with the don, even if in a way different from that of curers such as Lázaro and Manuela, whose midwives saw their don at their birth.

What we see in cases such as Martín's is that even someone not born with a physically discernible don can still later express an intuitive connection with bonesetting, one that can get further nourished by observing a bonesetter family member at work. Flavio thus talked about one of his sons who, even though he was not reportedly born with a don in his hand, was showing some talent at setting bones. "Since he was born, he knows," Flavio told me, pleased that his now eighteen-year-old son was learning. These skills should be kept up, he added, "so that it never dies."[15]

Expressions of Spiritual Osteopathology

Tz'utujiil Maya bonesetters pay attention to what the earth gives up because these revealed objects come to serve as vehicles of knowing. They extend the bonesetter's reach into the opaque spaces marked by injury, and they direct reparative influences to where they are most needed. When the baq enters the bonesetter's life—through the agency of other powers—the baq serves as a portal to realities deriving from outside of normal experience, amplifying the bonesetter's diagnostic senses when he or she places it on a body. But this quality of knowing and revealing is not limited to the baq, the bonesetters find. This property also belongs to the body itself, and more specifically to living bones in the body. Human bones, aside from supporting the body's weight and hosting cellular functions through the marrow, exercise important cultural functions for Mayas. Among Tz'utujiil Mayas we most often see this in relation to how Martín, Flavio, Raquel, and others struggle with pain and infirmity in the lead-up to accepting the bonesetting don. We get the sense that their own bones are forging channels of communication with their baq and with the bodies they treat. Elsewhere in the Maya area, bones also serve as conduits for important messages, sometimes even for spiritual messages. Tedlock (1992:57), for example, reports that in Momostenango, Guatemala, prospective K'iche' Maya calendar diviners are prone to a certain dislocation injury. The illness is called *k'ajinak bak* (dislocated bone) and is treated by a *wikol bak*. The curer bathes the affected area in a special herb, reduces the dislocation, wraps it in *tz'ite'* (*Erythrina corallodendron*) leaves, and sets it with *tz'ite'* splints. In this scenario, the victim is thought to be pushed, pulled, and sucked to the ground by the Mundo, a key earth lord.

Other kinds of spiritual aggressions register in the Tzotzil Maya body. Kevin Groark (2017) reported how a Tzotzil man in San Juan Chamula, Chiapas, experienced a musculoskeletal injury through a dream. In the man's dream, an envious neighbor in cat form attacked him, injuring the man's wrist (Groark 2017:321). For Tzotzils, according to Groark, dreams are an important stage through which local aggressions are played out, and these aggressions can leave a physical imprint. Dreams' significance stands out in earlier accounts of Tzotzil Mayas, as well. In San Andrés Larráinzar, Chiapas, Holland (1962:384–385) found that in some cases where a Tzotzil Maya was suffering severe bodily pain, it could be attributed to the person's dreams that his *chanul* (companion animal) had had its bones broken in fights with other animals or had been abused by *naguals* of the sacred mountain. Naguals are the familiars into which certain individuals transform themselves to attack others (Holland 1962: 143). A unique osteospiritual etiology thus unfolds for bodily injury and pain among these Mayas, one even extending to human spiritual counterparts and their bodies.

In these cases, the quality of the Maya body as a source of knowledge is heightened during moments of injury and debility. This aligns with how, as noted in chapter 2, Maya bonesetters whose bodies have suffered often have unique insights into other suffering bodies. Injury to the bones can be especially significant when the local culture recognizes spiritual causality in it, as in the K'iche' and Tzotzil cases, because treating the injury will involve both ritual and physical aspects. It is also significant that a person's spiritual component, such as the Tzotzil *chanul*, can be injured, causing suffering to its corresponding person. But though the osteospiritual dimension of bone injury and pain, with its supernatural etiology and treatment, appears in Maya bonesetting (Fabrega and Silver 1973; Paul 1976), it does not in Comalapa. For Kaqchikel bonesetters there, the supernatural carries little causative weight in the injuries they deal with or in the pains they themselves feel. They continue treating people with a very limited sense of the supernatural.

The Question of Status

As stated, among most Middle American bonesetters, supernatural approaches to work are deemphasized. This deemphasis of magicoreligious elements among most bonesetters, however, has produced certain consequences for them in terms of status. In the Maya region and greater Mexico, the work of bonesetters is often considered to be of rather low status when compared with other treatment specialties. This may be especially true in Mexico, where bonesetters are usually outnumbered by, and are younger than, other curers (Lozoya Legorreta et al. 1988:56; B. Paul and McMahon 2001:256). Mexican researchers identified this pattern when they examined Mexico's distribution of traditional curers, finding that those at the younger end of the scale, twenty and under, constituted a small percentage of the total number of curers and tended to be bonesetters and herbalists (Lozoya Legorreta et al. 1988:56). Their finding that practitioners of traditional medicine were predominantly over forty suggests in turn that young age can be a factor limiting one's status.[16]

Tzotzil Maya bonesetters of Larránzar, Chiapas, were likewise described as having rather low status among local curers (Holland 1962), but this had less to do with age than with other factors. In their case, even though their work contained supernatural elements, they tended to begin it out of an urgent need and not because of a ritual mandate. In addition, because they generally dealt with conditions that did not provoke as much anxiety as conditions dealt with by other curers, they enjoyed less status, according to Holland (1962:237). More recently, Nahuat bonesetters have been described as being of lower status than other curers in Hueyapan, Puebla (Huber and Anderson 1996), but this, too, may have to do more with how they work than with their age. Again, how curers begin their work, and whether curing specialists deploy magicoreligious operating methods, can mark those individual specialists as being higher or lower in status than others. To this effect, Huber and Anderson (1996:34) argue that Nahuat curers are afforded greater prestige than bonesetters because curers work in the spiritually charged realm of supernatural etiology, whereas bonesetters do not.

This status distinction operates even among bonesetters of a given place, as in the case of Zinacantan, Chiapas. There, according to Fabrega and Silver (1973:42), "the least highly regarded bonesetters are those who use actual physical manipulation of a broken or dislocated area—in short, a bonesetter who actually sets bones is considered inferior to one who merely prays over them." In local bonesetting, priority is given to healing by prayer over healing by manipulation. Curers who physically handle bones are considered less competent than those who do not. Among these Tzotzil Maya bonesetters, who Fabrega and Silver (1973:42) also assessed as "quite low" in number, the use of prayer brings a bonesetter higher status. The selective incorporation of magicoreligious elements was also found to upgrade the status of a Chorti' Maya massage specialist who performed otherwise manual therapy. Wisdom (1940:355) reported that Chorti' massagers normally did not use prayers and cured only "natural" ailments. But if a Chorti' massager wanted to make a strong impression on a client, he massaged the air above the client's body, invoking an imitative magic thought to be more effective than just rubbing. He accrued more prestige by using magic. The primacy of the physical in bonesetting and massage is greatly diminished in the Tzotzil and Chorti' cases, apparently with a corresponding diminishment in status.

In the Guatemalan highlands, the bonesetters' status can vary greatly from town to town. In some towns, they enjoy little notice and moderate status, whereas in others they enjoy a more pronounced public role and higher status. Their status, however, is not systematically higher or lower than that of other curers. In Comalapa, for example, there do not seem to be enormous status distinctions between Kaqchikel Maya bonesetters and other curers. On the other hand, in San Pedro La Laguna and San Juan La Laguna, Tz'utujiil Maya bonesetters enjoy a notably higher public status than do other curers. Features of the health landscape in each of these towns underlie this variability.

While Comalapan bonesetters are not completely eclipsed by other curers, they operate with less public notice and deal with fewer people than do curers like midwives. Since midwives are familiar with a wide range of health problems and perform a good deal of manual manipulation, they are considered somewhat more knowledgeable about health overall than bonesetters. This is especially the case since, as I discuss in the introduction, many midwives have undertaken some obligatory midwife training at local health facilities, and have sometimes also received health promoter training. Their involvement of a large measure of religiosity in their primary activities—prenatal massage and childbirth—likely contributes to the great public faith in them, as well.

The numerous bonesetters of San Pedro La Laguna and San Juan La Laguna, on the other hand, have created and kept a high public profile over the last few decades. Their skill at reducing dislocations and fractures has contributed greatly to their prestige, but their use of magico-religious elements has played an equally large role. By regularly using the baq, which is said to confer healing authority upon its owner, Tz'utujiil bonesetters bolster public confidence in them and attract more clients. San Pedro La Laguna, in particular, has become an especially strong draw for injured people and remains something of a prime Guatemalan destination for getting bones fixed.

Status differentials between bonesetters and other curers, and among bonesetters in a given community, can influence how individuals seek treatment for musculoskeletal problems. People naturally want to go with the practitioner who they think can best handle their problem, and a practitioner's higher status relative to his fellows can make the choice easier. This prompts many people in the lakeside towns to bring their injuries to the homes of bonesetters instead of to other curers. The relative status of a region's bonesetters can also prompt people to prefer bonesetters of one town over those of another, as in the case of San Pedro La Laguna. Comalapa residents, though, seem content with taking their musculoskeletal problems to local bonesetters rather than to out-of-town ones. They also seem to prefer taking their injuries to bonesetters rather than to other curers, such as midwives. Midwives might accept some minor injury cases (even though they are not known primarily for treating these). However, because treating many injury cases might be seen as activity outside their prescribed area of work, and because they are under regular surveillance by health authorities, they seem disinclined to accept more serious cases. To accept a major injury case could place their midwifery accreditation at risk, especially if a health center official were to learn of the nonmidwifery work. As a result, Comalapans regularly take their injury cases to bonesetters, less often to midwives, and still less often to physicians. The latter find this disconcerting, to say the least. But the space between formal and informal providers of care meandering through Maya communities is only one that people have learned to navigate. A closer look at bonesetters' experiences suggests that people have also learned to live with another societal division, one that cuts much closer to home.

Evangélico Experience and Bonesetting

Many Guatemalans consider themselves *evangélicos*, an identifier most often associated with strands of evangelical Protestantism that have flourished in the country since the late nineteenth century (Garrard-Burnett 1998). The term is sometimes applied to adherents of nonmainstream forms of Protestant Christianity as well (Stoll 1990:4, 103–104). Members of these groups all either personally converted from some form of traditionalist Catholicism, or they belong to families who converted a generation or two earlier. And it is in the process of converting and living an evangélico life that converts face tough choices about what to retain and discard from their preconversion life (Hinojosa 2018). But while these changes can have serious consequences for some expressions of Maya traditional medicine in the postconversion life, evangélicos' discernment of the worth of bonesetting gives the practice a durability that other traditions lack. Bonesetting has seemingly sidestepped the scrutiny directed at other forms of Maya traditional practice.

For example, many Maya converts and evangélicos disavow ritually centered traditionalist Maya practices, including those whose practitioners began through divine election. Evangelicals likewise often distance themselves from Maya healers whose work is anchored in ritual esoterica. Since the programs of evangelical congregations stress the need for converts to make a break from their past and accept salvation through Christ, many Maya evangélicos have felt compelled to reject all outward expressions of traditionalist thinking: participating in cofradías and town festivals, making offerings to the earth lords, drinking alcohol, and so forth (Annis 1987:79–80; Sexton 1978:294). They are also expected to stop subscribing to illnesses of spiritual etiology such as fright sickness and *mal de ojo* (a malady attributed to an invidious gaze), however challenging this may be.

Despite the changes that conversion experiences have produced in individuals and their communities, these changes have not been highly disruptive when it comes to Maya bonesetting. Most people regard bonesetting, like injury itself, in deeply pragmatic terms. When evangélicos get physically injured, they do not see this as having anything to do with church membership or spiritual etiology. Injury is a physical condition for which they need a physically skilled bonesetter. The bulk of bonesetters' work, as I have emphasized, is not considered to be ritual in nature, and even if it does utilize ritual, this is eclipsed by the predominately physical aspect of the work. Evangelicals therefore seem quite accepting of bonesetters, even in the Lake Atitlán area where there is a pronounced ritual aspect to many bonesetters' practices. As a result, people of different confessions seek bonesetters with little apparent regard for which church the bonesetters attend, if any. Moreover, because people in the lakeside towns participate in a common framework of revelation linked to the bonesetter role, people of various religious backgrounds become bonesetters in nearly identical ways and thereafter practice in ways more alike than different.

We can see how well the craft has fared in a few key instances in which evangélico bonesetters describe their formative experiences and in which a non-evangélico bonesetter treats evangélico clients. Their experiences showcase how bonesetters of a particular persuasion do not limit their work to others of that persuasion. Their work also tells us that Tz'utujiil Mayas do not typically view bonesetting through narrow congregational lenses, even if their bonesetting practice has spiritual underpinnings.

Consider Imelda, the bonesetter daughter of Martín. She stresses that as an *evangélica*, she does not use religious images or an altar. But in listening to her story, it is clear that what she credits as sparking her awareness of bonesetting is in line with what other local bonesetters experience. Imelda begins by saying that when she was a young woman she dreamed of a hueso. In this dream she also saw a rooster, which she took to be another *retal* (sign, omen) of some kind. At the time, she was Catholic, but this changed when she married an evangélico man and converted not long after. After getting married and converting, Imelda did some bonesetting work together with her husband, undeterred by the fact that she did not have a baq. But once they began their evangélico life and began working together, this changed. She went *pa juyu'* (to the hills/woods) one day and encountered a hueso. It was a unique stone in the form of a hand with five fingers and even knuckles. And though she picked it up that day, she did not start using it right away. It was around this time, she explains, that she became very sick. Still, she somehow knew that her sickness was yet another sign that *iba tener su trabajo* ([I] would have the work [of a bonesetter]).

Her narrative takes a curious turn here, I should note. On the one hand, she tells me that she had starting bonesetting when she got married, and basically continued doing it with a renewed sense of purpose after she found the hueso. After mentioning her sickness episode, though, she marks *that* as a definitive moment signaling her calling to bonesetting. This sickness episode, at any rate, seems to have reconfirmed the legitimacy of her calling, especially given that when she continued working (more diligently, apparently) as a curer, the sickness went away. Considering her narrative as a whole, Imelda bears witness to how she experienced divine election both *before* she converted to *evangelismo* (by dreaming of the hueso) and immediately *after* she converted to evangelismo (by finding the hueso, and getting sick and recovering). This narrative prompts two observations: (1) even though she downplays the visual emphasis of Catholicism and *costumbre*, she recognizes the authenticity of visual signs as experienced in her initial dream and in her eventual discovery of the hueso, and (2) Imelda's identity as an evangélica during the last two moments of divine election did nothing to dissuade her from accepting their sacred origin. To this day she carries her revealed hueso with her when she travels to other towns to treat people.

Raquel, a lifelong evangélica, also found herself being pulled toward the bonesetter role, but unlike Imelda she did not dream of a hueso; she simply found one. When she was small, she was playing in a coffee plantation and there it was. She collected it, admired it, and had her father put it away for her. When she got older, the hueso came into her possession again. But when she married and had her first child, some real problems began. For four or five years she struggled with sickness, and seemingly nothing she tried was helping. But one day a female acquaintance told her something she would never forget: "Usted tiene algo, usted tiene que curar" (There's something about you, you have to cure). The woman insisted to Raquel, "Usted es curadero [*sic*] del hueso. . . . Salí, o te vas a mantener así" (You are a bone curer. . . . Go [and treat others], or you will remain like you are). As Raquel tells me about what the woman said, she recalls that this woman had told her earlier that when Raquel got married, she should use the hueso to cure others. Before she got married she had never felt compelled to do any curing, but her attitude had changed. Once she began curing, her health problems cleared up. And even though she later suffered a rib and hip injury that a local *curandera* treated her for, Raquel fights through the pain she occasionally feels and receives people to treat.

We see with Raquel that her divine election unfolded in a sequence of events nearly identical to what traditionalist Mayas report: a revelation, a sickness experience, a guide telling her to accept the work, an acceptance of the work, and finally some relief from poor health and infirmity. Her evangélico outlook may have precluded her use of religious images or altars, but her awakening to the bonesetter role follows that of non-evangélico Mayas, people who do use religious images and altars. Evangélicas Raquel and Imelda keep busy as bonesetters because, before anything else, they are sought for and judged by their manual skills. The usual expectations of bonesetter qualifications apply to them, so they must use a revealed baq. And since they either transitioned into the bonesetting role or were confirmed in it following a bout of sickness, this deepened their sense of legitimacy and purpose for themselves, and no doubt in the eyes of others as well.

In common with other bonesetters, Lázaro treats whoever needs him without asking about church membership. He treats at least one evangélica churchgoer during a visit we make to Santiago Atitlán, an elderly woman whose painful hip he has been attending and who requests that he give her an injection of Reumetan. More interestingly, as we walk down an Atitlán street an evangélico pastor calls out to Lázaro, asking him to come to his house. The pastor, a local Tz'utujiil Maya, asks Lázaro to treat his arm. Lázaro enters his house, sits down with him, and examines his left arm. As he listens to the pastor describe his fall, he holds the injured arm and moves it gently. Then, as with any other client, Lázaro takes the baq from his pocket, kisses it, and applies it to the man's arm as his wife watches. When Lázaro is finished, he tells the pastor and his wife, who wears nontraditional dress, that he will return later in the week. The pastor thanks him, then takes some bills, and surreptitiously places them in Lázaro's hand as we walk out of the house. The pastor makes no attempt to conceal from his neighbors, however, the fact that the well-known Lázaro is attending to him, apparently not fearing censure.

Evangélico bonesetters no doubt operate in many highland towns. In Comalapa I have known two such bonesetters (Paulino and Rómulo), met a third (Tonia), and heard of one other. But as far as I know, in Comalapa no clergy of any kind issue injunctions against seeking care from bonesetters, like they do against seeking help from ritualists. This is because of the nearly completely secular brand of bonesetting found there.[17] But in the lakeside towns, where bonesetting traditions are freighted with spiritual significance, admonishments from clergy about seeking care from bonesetters would arguably be more likely, especially among Protestant and orthodox Roman Catholic churchgoers.[18] Clergy there would presumably disapprove of this expression of Maya spiritual life, even if it is embedded in a therapeutic tradition that directly and physically benefits people. Nonetheless, I have not heard of any such admonishments.

Does being an evangélico bonesetter, then, make any difference in terms of attracting or excluding clients? It is difficult to say. If a person is injured and the injury is severe, the tendency seems to be to take the person to the nearest, best-regarded bonesetter around, whether that bonesetter is evangélico or not. In Comalapa, especially, it seems also that if the injury is not considered severe, say, an ankle sprain, then the person's family might take more time to ponder which bonesetter to go to. If the family of the injured person is active in a particular temple, church, or prayer group, and they know a bonesetter in that group, they might prefer to seek that person's help. In this sense familiarity and perhaps proximity are important factors in choosing a bonesetter. But never have I heard of Comalapans choosing or avoiding certain bonesetters because those bonesetters are members of a particular religious group. The bonesetter's practical abilities are the overriding concern.

The situation in San Pedro La Laguna and San Juan La Laguna is not so different from that of Comalapa in this respect. In the lakeside towns, injured people also tend to be brought to bonesetters who are established and well regarded. If they are known to the family of the injured and live nearby, this is a plus. But while some families may decide to consult particular bonesetters because those bonesetters are members of their religious group, this does not seem to be the most important consideration when choosing a practitioner. Again, a bonesetter's general reputation is far more important. In addition, as the examples from the lake area bonesetters suggest, the experience of bonesetting may be so deeply woven into the fabric of San Pedro La Laguna and San Juan La Laguna life that the church with which a bonesetter identifies is of little consequence when it comes to choosing a curer.

It is also the case that in these Tz'utujiil Maya communities a bonesetter's reputation hinges on more than just his or her perceived success rate; it hinges on whether or not he or she operates with divine sanction. This in turn means that bonesetters in the lakeside towns view each other more as rivals than as colleagues. A similarly tense state of affairs, though without supernatural overtones, exists among bonesetters of Comalapa, suggesting that bonesetting is overall more fraught with internal tensions than has been previously recognized.

The Don, the Authentic, and Noncollegiality

Mayas in Guatemala talk about bonesetters, and they sometimes wonder aloud whether certain bonesetters have got what it takes to work. But whether they learn about those bonesetters by interacting with them, by seeing their results, or just by hearing about them, over time they develop a sense of what makes a bonesetter genuine. They also notice when certain bonesetters seem to be lacking in something. In this context people often single out curers for either having or not having a validating gift, basically claiming that not all practicing bonesetters are really qualified to be bonesetters. Bonesetters make these claims about other bonesetters, too, revealing something of the deep tensions already in place among them. Comments by bonesetters about who is or is not qualified to work further stoke these tensions and do little to encourage any sense of joint purpose or collegiality among them. We see instead a thickening climate of suspicion enfolding many Maya bonesetters and their publics, one that threatens to erode the tenuous trust that has until now held between them.

When people assert who is qualified to work, they do so according to the validating criteria that operate in individual places. In Comalapa, for example, one often hears something to the effect of "so-and-so doesn't really know how to cure," or "so-and-so's cures don't last." The implication is that those persons lack the hand-based knowledge that local bonesetting values. In San Pedro La Laguna and San Juan La Laguna, on the other hand, a reproach usually sounds like "so-and-so doesn't have a don," or "so-and-so doesn't have a baq," speaking to how having a divinely conferred gift affects the bonesetter's authenticity there. Although the bonesetters' hands must know the body well in both Comalapa and the lakeside towns, because there is a more developed sense of validating criteria for bonesetters in the lakeside towns, residents there have a lot more to say about this. They appreciate a show of skill by bonesetters, but this is not enough. These specialists still need to have the right credentials.

This is clearly on Magda's mind when she tells me that a certain man in San Pedro La Laguna treats people without using a hueso. She insists that he does not cure well, because without a hueso, "no se cura, solo se hincha" (it doesn't get cured, it just swells). Lacking a revealed hueso, then, he is bound to get poor results. Lázaro, meanwhile, takes a more principled stand on bonesetter validation. He tells me that some people in San Pedro La Laguna practice bonesetting without even a don. Lacking the "don de Dios" (God's gift), he says, for them bonesetting is just a business. But while much of his indignation stems from how these presumably illegitimate bonesetters may charge sixty to a hundred quetzals per treatment (Lázaro accepts around ten quetzals per treatment), he implies that they might even be using a baq in their ill-starred practice, and this agitates him even more. As someone who believes strongly in the don and in one of its materializations, the baq, Lázaro considers these to be important marks of the true bonesetter.

But having the don or a baq does not guarantee respect from the community or from other bonesetters. Nor has it shielded Lázaro himself from suspicion. One of Victorino's young granddaughters tells me about a man who lives where the dead are (i.e., the cemetery) who uses a hueso but who still does not know how to cure. She then names Lázaro as this man. Raising a complaint sometimes voiced about some bonesetters, she then says that Lázaro charges a lot, much more than the one-quetzal fee that her grandfather Victorino charges. Although she has surely heard a lot about local bonesetters by living in Victorino's house, and though she is close to her grandfather, she sounds earnest in her criticism of Lázaro. She even makes me wonder just how much bonesetters talk about each other and compare themselves with each other.

I get part of my answer from Damiana, a woman from San Pedro La Laguna who sells weavings in the lakeside commercial center, Panajachel. When I tell her I am speaking with bonesetters in her hometown, she scoffs, saying that many who claim to be bonesetters there are not really bonesetters at all. Damiana says that she, on the other hand, knows how to set bones, and as she speaks with me she positions her index fingers point-to-point at eye level and explains that she can *feel* when bones are out of line, that she can *feel* the broken tips of bones. Just why she stresses this becomes clearer when I mention that many bonesetters in San Pedro La Laguna have found a hueso. She does not have a hueso and does not need one, she retorts, adding that even those people who have a hueso do not know how to heal with them. "Es mentira ante Dios" (It is a lie before God), she states, pointing to the sky. Damiana has the don and this is what matters, she insists, not whether or not she has a hueso. She does not mince words.

A few main points emerge if we consider these views. First, no matter the town, a bonesetter is never fully above suspicion. Other locals, bonesetters or otherwise, might take issue with a bonesetter's way of working. Second, and particularly in the lake area, suspicion is likely to fall on those bonesetters thought to not have the don or to not use a baq. These points tie in to stated Tz'utujiil Maya expectations of bonesetting, and set the stage for an important caveat I consider the third point: even if one has the don and its material expression, the baq, one's legitimacy can still be undermined by charging too much. Neighbors hear neighbors talking about who charges what, and even if a bonesetter has excellent results or comes from a family with accomplished bonesetters, there are limits to remuneration. Bonesetting comes from a gift, after all, and should be shared if not freely, at least with a sense of modesty.

Not all lakeside residents hold these views, of course, and people think differently about whether one needs the don, or the don and a baq, to work. But residents of San Pedro La Laguna and San Juan la Laguna still convey the sense that they know more about bonesetting than anyone else. Paul (1976:77) even mentioned how injured people came from all around Guatemala to see San Pedro La Laguna's bonesetters, something that probably suffused local bonesetting with a great deal of confidence. Speaking to the sense that the Tz'utujiil bonesetters' brand of care is the most authentic are depictions of bonesetters that have found their way into public spaces. One such depiction is prominently displayed in mural form in San Juan La Laguna. And the stated reason for this bonesetting authenticity is, again, the revealed baq. Victorino's daughter, Magda, says as much when I tell her that the bonesetters I know in San Juan Comalapa do not use the hueso. After first expressing surprise that there are curanderos in Comalapa in the first place, she shakes her head and says that curing without the hueso is not good. Apart from her claim that bonesetters fail to achieve good physical results without the hueso, she tells me that to cure without the hueso "just isn't right."

She does not outright berate Comalapan bonesetters, but she does not have to. Most bonesetters from the lakeside towns see their way of bonesetting—anchored in a don, dreams, and a revealed object—as making a lot of sense, much more sense, at any rate, than bonesetting traditions that lack these things. This prizing of the local by Tz'utujiil bonesetters, though, threatens to obscure a larger reality enveloping bonesetters throughout Guatemala. Commonalities of caring for others aside, bonesetters do not see much in common with each other. Whether in a local setting or across the region, they do not speak of each other as colleagues or as equals. They see each other somewhat as rivals, and at times one can detect more than a hint of animosity between them. During the episode I described at the start of the book, in which Lázaro hid from the other bonesetter knocking at the door, I glimpsed some of the lengths to which bonesetters will go to avoid other bonesetters in a care setting. It was not something I expected to see, especially since I knew both of the bonesetters involved. But though it was hard making sense of that moment at the time, I later understood it as part of a spectrum of avoidance- and disparagement-driven behaviors bonesetters take part in. It was one expression of disquiet in an environment of tension enfolding many bonesetters and their clients.

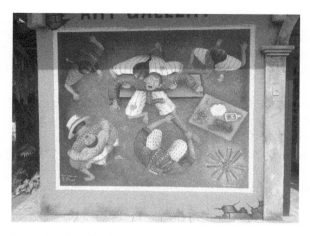

Figure 3.9. Mural in San Juan La Laguna depicting a bonesetter at work, 2012. The bonesetter holds a baq in his left hand. Note that the treatment appears to be taking place in a public, market-like environment and that a man is carrying a boy with a bandaged right leg, perhaps awaiting his turn. Photo courtesy of Mirela Conner.

One outcome of this noncollegiality is that even if a bonesetter has reached the limits of her or his abilities, she or he will not send clients to other bonesetters. They retain an abiding suspicion about other bonesetters, and to this day I do not know of any bonesetters who refer clients to each other. I have seen bonesetters act with some equanimity toward one another only when bonesetters have first-degree relatives who are bonesetters, such as when an older bonesetter has children who are also bonesetters or who are becoming bonesetters. We see this with Victorino and Martín and some of their adult children. As for why these related bonesetters temper their professional feelings toward each other, there are two main reasons. For the elder bonesetters, we might say it behooves them to recognize skill in their children, especially since their children have learned primarily from watching them, and because these elders may have even given their revealed baq to their child. Having their children perform well, or at least saying that they perform well, reflects well on the elders.

In the case of adult children who are setting bones, there is something else at work, too. One can sense deference to the bonesetter parent, something that might even prompt the younger bonesetter to work with less severe cases while leaving the more severe cases to the parent. For Imelda, Martín's daughter, this meant that she treated only small children during the time her father was still alive. Only after his death, when she was no longer in her father's shadow, did she begin developing a broader client base. Javier, Victorino's son, has also found it possible to treat more people and to come into his own after his father died. And as with his sister Magda, his status as Victorino's child affords him a good measure of legitimacy.

As the children of bonesetters, though, Imelda, Javier, and Magda will have to do more than just prove themselves able workers. They will have to live up to the reputation of their parents, and this might be too much for them. It is one thing to have a don and a revealed baq, but to be the standard-bearers of their well-known fathers may prove to be something else entirely. They might find this to be too demanding and time consuming in the end, and to leave them with too little room to generate the income their families need. Things might change by the time they reach middle age, but for now they work as best as they can under their fathers' shadows, relying only on themselves.

They will have to rely on themselves because by all accounts, and even though they work in ways that might seem to be more alike than different, Maya bonesetters remain untethered to a common identity. Bonesetters lack the group identity and collegiality that increasingly characterize the experience of Maya midwives, who find themselves beset by the health system and having to demand more recognition of it, as I discussed in the introduction. The midwives' ability to nurture a group identity in the face of an often contemptuous health establishment has enabled them to increasingly take action as a group. But to the extent that bonesetters may appear relatively weak against the health establishment or legal systems, and lack a coherent group identity, it is important to stress that their work germinated outside of and has remained outside of biomedical contexts. They were never pulled into the orbit of the health system as midwives were. The bonesetters' work has likewise remained outside of legal contexts. Since the bonesetters' work does not eventuate in a reality needing legal documentation (e.g., a newborn child), they have not been pressed in the way midwives have to get formal recognition as practitioners and, thus, to develop the legalistic acumen that midwives have increasingly had to exhibit.

Another important reality affecting the ability of midwives to kindle a group identity, organize themselves, and present a unified front to the Ministry of Public Health resides in the international domain. A proliferation of international actors and agencies have visited, worked with, or otherwise endorsed Maya midwives in Guatemala, affording them a degree of international visibility and credibility that bonesetters simply do not have (Berry 2006:1963; Cosminsky 2016:220–224). Many North American and European midwifery organizations, for instance, arrange for their members either to carry out training rotations with affiliated Guatemalan groups or to directly train Guatemalan midwives in those groups (see Julajuj 2017b). Guatemalan midwives have often leveraged this credibility to draw attention to their needs, and their international partners and funders have carried their cause far beyond the borders of the country (World Bank 2017). Getting actively sought and recruited by these well-organized groups has likely promoted a deeper sense of validation among midwives, something that has in turn bolstered their group identity and their basis for organizing around a common purpose.

These conditions mean midwives are far better positioned than bonesetters to engender a cohesive identity, to act on it, and to build an organized front against government agents. Bonesetters, moreover, find themselves working in arenas accorded less importance by health authorities and, lacking a basis for recognizing their fellows, have subsequently been unable to forge a sense of joint purpose with them. Absent the international endorsement that midwives enjoy, furthermore, any basis for organizing among bonesetters is further diluted. Without any significant changes on these unique fronts, the prospects for organizing by bonesetters remain extremely slim.

With these considerations in mind, I reiterate that a key reason bonesetters do not organize themselves or identify as a formal group ties back to the very reason why bonesetters are not as amenable to biomedical programs as are midwives: the physical and legal/bureaucratic realities of their respective work. Midwives work in a legally bounded activity, and so they must cooperate with health and civil authorities. Their mandated cooperation with health centers requires that they train and work in cohorts, which in turn makes their practice outcomes more documented and more visible to those international actors interested in further supporting and organizing them. Neither of these conditions applies to bonesetters or their work.

Comparing the situation of Maya bonesetters with that of corporate groups provides another way to frame the bonesetters' weak basis for organizing. If we consider Michael G. Smith's (1955, 1974) discussions of corporate groupings, we can appreciate how most of the groups to which he attributes a corporate character organize in terms of unilineal descent and make claims on group resources on this basis. The corporate group, often tied to a territory, performs many administrative duties for its members and represents the group among other like groups, indeed acting as a legal individual (Keesing 1975:17). These characteristics, however, present a scenario distinct from what we see among Maya bonesetters. They are not tied to a group identity organized around a common principle of descent, and they make no claims as bonesetters over any group material resources. Having no joint holdings, they lack the means to collectively mobilize when faced with common concerns. The shared material resources that figure prominently in Smith's (1955, 1974) formulations of corporate groups are here unavailable to foster any group identity. Bonesetters' lives go unregulated by the strictures of an organized collective, and bonesetters have shown no interest in or capacity for resolving disputes as a group. They mobilize no "machinery for mediation" in this respect, as Smith (1974:87) puts it. Last, they lack the ability to act as an administrative unit, undermining what Smith (1955:64) sees as key to a group's corporate character. Overall, we do not see bonesetters cleaving to a group identity, organizing, or mobilizing group resources in any tangible, much less corporate, manner.

Lest we restrict the possibility of corporate character only to groups that claim descent from an apical ancestor, organize as a single unit, and manage joint holdings, however, we would do well to note that Smith (1974:84–85) further explains that *occupations* can serve as an organizing principle for a corporate unit, referring to "trade unions," "professional associations," and other groupings. In these collectives members work largely according to the rules and stipulations set forth by their groups. To the extent that healers might also form such associations, it stands to reason that they would have to work as much by the terms set by their group as by an abiding interest in meeting the individual needs of their clients. Arguably, they might even be expected to subordinate the individual needs of their clients to the work requirements of their professional group. This would result in a situation in which healers who are organized in a corporate manner would not be able to operate fully independently of their group strictures.

Here, too, though, do we see incongruence with the Maya bonesetter case. The Maya healers I discuss emphasize that their individual ways of working produce results and, by implication, that the ways other bonesetters work do not. They neither train nor advance in skill together, and express no solidarity that might plant the seeds of a unified syndicate or legal front among them. But though Maya bonesetters are not constrained by corporate group strictures as such, they do have to act in accord with expectations set by the local practitioner group (i.e., having a don and a baq; relying on hands and not X-rays). So while bonesetters may adhere, albeit informally, to certain group expectations, these still reveal nothing to indicate that their outlook is a collective one. This contextualizes how, even though the World Health Organization encourages its partners and stakeholders to "foster cohesiveness among traditional health practitioners and empower them to organize into associations or groups,"[19] current conditions are not conducive to this among Maya bonesetters in Guatemala.

Licensing and Its Prospects

In view of their weak basis for recognizing a common identity or even a store of knowledge that could be systematized by the health system, neither does it appear likely that training and licensing will be possible for bonesetters anytime soon. As it is, they face little acknowledgment, much less recognition, from the health system. For there to be an institutional basis for training and licensing bonesetters, there would first need to be clear agreement among clinicians that this is the right way forward. Instead, key voices point out either the restrictions that bonesetter training would entail, the impracticalities of training bonesetters, or the ethical problems that could follow the licensing of bonesetters.

Much of this discussion emerges when physicians talk about what it would mean to train curers in general and to license bonesetters in particular. When Dr. Cun, of Comalapa, talks about curers, for example, he likes the idea of training them. But he says that above all, curers should be trained to identify sicknesses and to know when these sicknesses are too critical for them to handle. Their training and their ability to know their limitations should be established as a matter of policy, he says. Dr. Sotz', of Comalapa, seems to agree that this is the right course of action, and while he feels, hypothetically, that bonesetters can be trained, he looks at it from the point of view of logistics. To properly train bonesetters, he says, one would have to first identify who is going to do the trainings. One would then have to create a training methodology, and after this those who are going to be trained would have to be identified. It is a big task, he muses, and says that there is simply no time to do it. He does not see this training as a pathway to a license, at any rate.

When I asked Laura, an administrator at ASECSA, whether bonesetters could be trained and licensed, meanwhile, she also turned to a core issue of health system limitations: she indicated that bonesetters "don't use or qualify for any (current) assigned certifications." They are unlike midwives in this way, who do have a certification available to them that permits them to operate openly and that forms the basis for knowledge exchanges through ASECSA. In other words, since bonesetter knowledge has not yet been formalized to the point that it can be didactically taught, no framework for testing can be formulated. And without a testing framework, the licensing question is moot.

As we can see, whether or not these individuals agree that training and licensing curers such as bonesetters is a good idea, or even feasible, they harbor many reservations about it. For the most part, they do not see any real prospects for it. These views probably reflect, among other things, a limited understanding of how bonesetters work and how their work outcomes cannot be measured by the same scales used for midwives' work outcomes. They also reflect a pervasive medical disquiet about bonesetting.

It thus comes as little surprise that when I ask Dr. Hugo Icú Perén of ASECSA about whether bonesetters can be trained, he replies, "Lo veo difícil, difícil" (In my view, this would be very, very hard). Part of the problem, according to him, goes back to the bonesetters themselves. He says that getting them into a training setting "depende un poco (de) que tanta cancha pueden dar" (depends somewhat on how much of a chance the bonesetters will give [for this]). Because Maya bonesetters *son duros* (are a tough crowd), he is not sure they would even come to a training. As for issuing bonesetters a license to practice, Dr. Icú Perén is equally pessimistic, reiterating, "Yo lo miro muy, muy difícil, no imposible, pero difícil" (I see this as extremely difficult, not impossible, but difficult). He adds, "En relación a componehuesos yo pienso que estamos muy lejos" (In terms of [training] bonesetters I believe we're still a long way off). Even if he could arrange such a training program, he says that another formidable problem could arise, this time with physicians. He admits, "La parte del carnet, tendría que ser . . . los traumatólogos [que lo den], y no creo que suelten" (As for the license, it would have to be the traumatologists who issue it, and I don't think they're going to yield this up). With this acknowledgment that physicians themselves would oppose bonesetter training and licensing, he signals how the medical establishment remains very reluctant to validate nonbiomedical practitioners by issuing them credentials.

In the case of this physician, we have a medical professional who feels strongly that it is unfeasible to try to locate, train, and license bonesetters. His voice carries particular weight because not only does the organization he leads make it a point to identify, interact with, and value practitioners of traditional medicine, but in his own 1990 medical thesis—which was about Maya bonesetters—he initially argued that bonesetters *should* seek a license to practice. He says now, though, that he made this argument back when he was an inexperienced young physician; he has since moved away from the idea that bonesetters should seek licensure.

In fact, he now feels that with "traditional therapists"— bonesetters, midwives, herbalists, and others—"más urge una protección que someterlos a un cuadro oficial" (it's more important to protect them than to submit them to an official framework). This has been a major problem in the case of midwives, who have submitted to training and who have received a permit to practice (a *carnet*), because they have routinely suffered discrimination and mistreatment in clinical settings and have seen many limitations placed on their work. Consequently, Dr. Icú Perén is wary of what can happen when traditional healers get certification. Referring again to midwives, he says, "Hay un debate que el carnet de comadrona no sea de abuso" (People are talking about how the midwives' carnet shouldn't be a way to mistreat them). He does not want to repeat with bonesetters the missteps taken with midwives, namely, the way the health system licensed them and then opened the door to delimiting and maltreating them. Laura, the administrator at ASECSA, who works closely with midwives, agrees. For her it is clear that "cuando empezaron a organizar a las comadronas, empezaron a violar sus derechos" (when [the health system] began to organize midwives, they began to infringe on their rights). Trainings and certifications speak more in her view to the health system's need for control than to any affirmation of native knowledge. As a result, says Dr. Icú Perén, there should be great caution going forward.

He worries, for this reason, about what might happen with bonesetters if they, however unlikely, were to receive licenses to practice, because the licenses would surely come at a great cost to their knowledge and autonomy. As it now stands, his organization tries to encourage traditional medicine specialists to talk with each other, a task he performs with great care, "pa' tratar de no invadir [su trabajo]" (to avoid invading [their work]). To license bonesetters would accelerate a biomedical intrusion into the very kind of work his organization is trying to buffer from external control. The bonesetters' work, an arena that has until now been largely free of clinical oversight, would probably see its operating space shrink dramatically, as well as witness other changes. Based on what she has seen happen with midwives, Laura argues of Maya bonesetters that "si están certificados, serían controlados" (if they [were] licensed, they would be overseen/controlled) by health officials. Dr. Icú Perén agrees that such changes would not be of any benefit to Maya bonesetting, and would instead embolden the Ministry of Public Health to extend its already long reach into the lives of ordinary Guatemalans.

Still, in the absence of licensing, the question of what the ministry intends to do regarding bonesetters, if anything, goes unanswered. Unlike with midwives, who are ostensibly prohibited from practicing if they are not trained and certified, there is no protocol in place concerning bonesetters. This leaves open whether the ministry as a whole or individual health center jurisdictions might try to restrict the bonesetters' work in some way. While it is possible that the health system might formalize its grievances with bonesetters and take restrictive action against them, there are no indications that this is happening. The health system remains opaque about this. As it currently stands, then, even though clinicians routinely cast aspersions on bonesetters, and even though they do not agree on whether bonesetters can be trained, the health system itself has not made clear how it will interact with bonesetters, leaving them in uncertain territory.

So while tensions exist between clinicians and bonesetters, these do not currently rise to the level of legal confrontation. It is unclear what the health system would stand to gain from such a confrontation, at any rate. Any actions of this kind would probably deepen popular resentment against it, something that could alienate more users than it would attract. For this reason a particular WHO document is worth mentioning. In a 2001 report about the legal status of traditional medicine, the organization refers to how traditional-medicine practitioners in Guatemala might get sued for malpractice.[20] It leaves out specifics about the grounds for such lawsuits, but it still implies that an atmosphere of latent litigiousness operates in the country, presumably in the rural areas where curers are especially active. Even if the report is referring primarily to midwives, who can be somewhat reprimanded if they work without a certificate to practice, the prospect of lawsuits is still hard to square with daily reality. Never have I heard of health officials actually suing midwives or bonesetters, nor have I heard of a looming threat to do so. Whatever legal urgency is alluded to in the report seems to exist more on paper than on the street, and at least for now, bonesetters continue working largely free of legal entanglements.

For the foreseeable future, then, bonesetters can expect to work in an environment that has yet to act in an official capacity toward them. They can also expect to work without the support of other bonesetters and without the conditional authority of a license. Maya bonesetters will instead continue helping others like generations of bonesetters have done before them: relying mostly on themselves and, if they live by Lake Atitlán, relying on the little baq that the Earth saw fit to grant them. Bonesetters in the three communities can also foresee working in a world increasingly permeated by newer technologies. But while some of these technologies have presented real challenges to the bonesetters' work, many bonesetters have responded to them in ways both novel and telling, as the next chapter reports.

CHAPTER 4

Challenges and Changes
in the Injury Landscape

When it comes to treating musculoskeletal problems in Guatemala, people seem to prefer bonesetters over physicians. For this reason, bonesetters, according to their level of skill and reputation, see a steady stream of clients. But this has dismayed many physicians in Maya communities, who feel they alone should receive trauma cases. Part of this situation stems from the physicians' lack of familiarity with body-centered ways of working, but a large part also stems from matters of professional status with which physicians themselves wrestle. In the end, by reiterating what does and does not constitute legitimate body care, each kind of practitioner plays a large role in defining the other. And with the entry of more urban resources into rural areas, the possibilities for contrasting the legitimacy of physicians and bonesetters have grown still further.

Recent decades have seen radiography expand into the places where Maya bonesetters practice, and this has directly impacted their work. This element of biotechnology is clearly affecting how bonesetters, their clients, and biomedical workers size up injury and even how they regard each other. What is unclear is how the bonesetting craft will respond to this outside technology over the long term, or even if it can survive it. The future of Maya bonesetting may hinge as much upon how bonesetters manage the growing availability of X-rays as it does on how it handles the more immediate pressure of living in the crosshairs of biomedicine. Bonesetters' and physicians' views of each other's qualifications can help illustrate this.

Engagement between Maya Bonesetters and Biomedicine

The ability to sense another person's injury using one's own body and to detect supernatural agency at work upon bodies is needed for healing legitimacy among Maya bonesetters. Physicians practicing biomedicine, however, have to neither perceive with their bodies nor be conversant in spiritual etiology. Bonesetters do, and this has had an unsettling effect on the physicians I spoke with. So while Maya people tend to have great confidence in the abilities of bonesetters, the bonesetters' diagnostic and therapeutic methods have been questioned by those with little understanding of their modus operandi, physicians. Bonesetters, in turn, express doubt about the physicians' abilities, particularly when it comes to treating musculoskeletal problems.

Maya bonesetters argue that physicians mishandle fractures, and they often talk about this. "They simply put casts on them," bonesetters usually claim when asked about the physicians' treatment of broken bones. Bonesetters contend that physicians do not or cannot use their hands to probe the fracture, identify its constituent elements, or realign the bones. Rather, the physicians simply cover the injury and let the bones mend however they will. To make matters worse, according to bonesetters and other Mayas, physicians do not periodically remove the immobilizing devices they apply to breaks to verify that the alignment is holding, thereby neglecting to perform the kind of visual and manual reexamination of the injury that bonesetters consider absolutely critical. Bonesetters worry that if they do not check the injury site regularly a problem might develop and go undetected. The bones might come out of alignment and not knit properly, resulting in deformity or immobility. Bonesetters say that even with the aid of X-rays, physicians have difficulty aligning bones and keeping them aligned. For reasons stemming from their own experience, then, bonesetters do not consider physicians proficient in fracture care. They do feel, though, that physicians can handle other problems such as fevers, open wounds, and some fractures requiring surgery. But since in some communities there seem to be fewer and fewer Maya bonesetters who accept fracture cases (see later in this chapter), fracture sufferers will increasingly need to resort either to a physician or to a Maya bonesetter in another town.

Bonesetters thus find value in the work physicians do, but say that their abilities have limits. Most physicians, on the other hand, refuse to recognize any abilities among bonesetters or to concede any legitimacy to them. Seven of the nine physicians I spoke with in Comalapa, San Pedro La Laguna, and Panajachel either dismiss the bonesetters' knowledge and abilities outright or speak rather ambivalently about them. In their official capacity, physicians take issue with how Maya bonesetters are untrained in Western trauma treatment and might cause irreparable harm to people's bodies. And even though in Guatemala many medical personnel assigned to government health posts in rural areas have limited experience in treating musculoskeletal injury, as a physician in rural practice reports (Acevedo Ligorria 1986:109), physicians readily talk about how a given person was injured, went to a bonesetter for help, and was left with a permanent limp or deformity.

Most of the time, however, physicians quietly tolerate popular bonesetting, much as they must also accept the work of midwives, a certain degree of which still falls outside their purview. In a way, physicians accept their postings to government health centers knowing that they have very little experience not only with pregnancy and childbirth but with dislocations and fractures, injuries befalling many people in rural areas.

Physicians are further troubled by what they have heard about the bonesetters' hand-based knowledge, questioning the very idea of it and arguing that bonesetters should not handle broken bones, with or without any special skills. The bonesetters' claims of hand-based knowledge moreover leave physicians unsettled and puzzled. In the words of Comalapan physician Dr. Sisimit, "Like the [bonesetters] say, it's a, it's a . . . it's something that they have . . . it's a *don* [gift] to them." As to whether this physician would himself reduce fractures the way bonesetters do, he says, "I wouldn't *dare* do it . . . do it like that empirically." By "empirically," he means without the relatively sophisticated technology, such as radiographic imaging, on which local physicians rely heavily. And because bonesetters do not rely on this technology, various physicians say, the bonesetters' approach to treatment is also inherently flawed. For Dr. Arana, in San Pedro La Laguna, the bonesetter's reliance on his or her hands (instead of X-rays) creates a situation in which "every pain is treated as though it were a fracture," at once suggesting that bonesetters cannot distinguish between different types of injuries and that they are overly eager to manually work the body. As a result, says Dr. Sotz', the attending physician at Comalapa's Health Center, when bonesetters treat injured people, "they make them worse; [patients] arrive here mishandled." But the damage does not stop there. According to Dr. Cun, of Comalapa, even the ways bonesetters immobilize bones *after* treatment makes the fractures worse, given that they have only their hands to guide them. After sharing similar frustrations about bonesetters, and offering accounts of bonesetter treatments gone wrong, Dr. Vélez, of Panajachel, remarks, "It's awful what those *sobadores* do."

Other declarations by physicians reveal their disdain not just for how bonesetters rely on their hands, but for the products bonesetters use or are thought to use. Dr. Suárez, of Comalapa, for instance, who otherwise says that bonesetters attend to fractures quite well, tempers this positive assessment by claiming that when bonesetters treat people, "they get them drunk [first]." Some medical specialists take issue with other materials bonesetters might use on injured people. Dr. Icú Perén, of Comalapa, says that clinicians scold people who they think have been massaged by a bonesetter. A clinician might chastise a patient "because he smells of leaves" that a bonesetter supposedly applied and demand to know "who touched you?!" Aligning himself closely with how these clinicians view bonesetters, Dr. Arana, meanwhile, concludes that "the people believe blindly in them, precisely because of the traditions deriving from their ancestors." Even Dr. Suárez, who tries to see bonesetters in a more positive light, sympathizes with Dr. Arana's view, remarking of the many people who go to curers, "No salen de sus costumbres" ([These people] don't get out of their native ways of being). At least a couple of the physicians I spoke with, then, imply that Maya care-seekers are trapped in their ancestral ways, as shown by their acceptance of bonesetters. Other physicians simply shake their heads when describing how people continue seeking bonesetters instead of medical care. Unable to abide this misplaced trust, but knowing that people in remote areas have little choice but to go to bonesetters, Comalapa's Dr. Sucuc, who happens to be Maya, states simply, "I can speak neither well nor ill of them." The positions many physicians take on bonesetters might also be influenced, I should note, by reports that some bonesetters learned their craft by treating animals.[1]

The way community physicians size up bonesetters is, moreover, bound up in the fact that these physicians consider themselves to be working on a professional periphery in rural practice and, therefore, as greatly needing to elevate their professional status. There is a hierarchy among Guatemalan physicians, and rural physicians often complain that they are seen by their urban counterparts as "public health" physicians, relegated to the low-status end of medicine. Their social construction of themselves in the rural areas usually involves an ongoing critique of traditional healers, especially of those healers — bonesetters and midwives, for example — who are called to intervene in situations that physicians feel themselves solely qualified to handle.

Ironically, as Robert Anderson (1983) has noted, since the eighteenth century European and North American health practitioners who use physical manipulation (e.g., osteopaths and chiropractors) have been stigmatized and considered low status by other health practitioners. This finding could be understood more broadly to suggest that among biomedical practitioners, a disdain exists for things of rural-folk extraction and for practices such as bonesetting descended from such rural-folk traditions. That Comalapa physicians would aspire to skills in traumatology and orthopedics, given Anderson's observation, suggests that these specialties have not yet been practiced long enough in Guatemala for them to be overshadowed and eclipsed in status by other medical specialties. As it now stands, medical fracture reduction is seen by physicians as a step up from mere "public health" status, and this appeals to them.

Well aware of how they are regarded by physicians, bonesetters limit their contact with them. Physicians likewise tend to keep their distance from bonesetters and other traditional healers. But in the process, each practitioner builds up an image of a practitioner-self partially by talking about members of the other group and about his or her fellows. As I have explained earlier, though, bonesetters do not view themselves as a group in the same way that physicians do; they do not think of themselves as a harmonious, allied whole positioned against the medical establishment. Even though bonesetters feel that, as individuals, they do better work than physicians, they do not speak of each other as team members or colleagues in the way that physicians or, increasingly, Maya midwives, do. Yet just as physicians rank themselves against other physicians, bonesetters often speak of the poor abilities or poor track records of other bonesetters. What is more, they often do this by likening another bonesetter to a physician, someone who, in their opinion, mishandles clients' injuries and causes the client to go to a second bonesetter for corrective help.

Although physicians retain a tighter organizational structure than do bonesetters (who have no structure to speak of), they are at a loss when it comes to dealing with bonesetters, in contrast to how they feel about dealing with midwives. As I discuss in the introduction, clinicians generally agree that the health system should use Maya midwives to provide health services and products to as many Maya households as possible (Hinojosa 2004a; Maupin 2008). And though the logic of this view has been scrutinized (Jordan 1993), it prevails in Guatemala. On the other hand, there is little sense among physicians that bonesetters can provide an effective "window of access" into the community in the way midwives can.[2] This being the case, providing bonesetters with trainings and granting them licenses to practice, as is done with Guatemalan midwives, remains both impractical and untenable at present, as I explain in chapter 3.[3] An adversarial view of bonesetters solidifies, as shown by the way physicians talk about bonesetters. This extends even to local physicians who are themselves Maya.

The importance of Maya bonesetting has been obscured by the resulting fraught atmosphere kept in place by medical workers, who eschew the main tenets of bonesetting. The element of bonesetting under the most scrutiny, the application of hand-based knowledge, is of key interest here. Maya bonesetting is predicated on the somatic availability of information, something underpinning the bonesetters' ability to directly apprehend the problems of the suffering body. This direct engagement with the body threatens to obviate the need for diagnostic technologies and allows the client to receive low-cost treatment. The medical injunction against the therapeutic handling of bodies by "unschooled" persons is thus emblematic of how the medical establishment prioritizes instrumentation over manipulation, favors diagnostic radiographs over diagnostic palpation, and promotes perfunctory casting over careful immobilization. It also speaks to how community physicians wish to increase their professional status by delegitimizing indigenous providers of manual medicine. I am reminded of Gemma Burford et al.'s (2007:368) observation that among Nigerian physicians, it has become something of a fashion to decry the work of Nigerian traditional bonesetters and to overlook the range of services they provide. Physicians in Guatemala, similarly, take the view that since bonesetter body manipulation is not taught by formal didactic methods, it must be illegitimate. It can even provoke strong reactions among physicians—recall how Dr. Hugo Icú Perén said that clinicians might ask a person treated by a bonesetter, "Who touched you?!" And even if bonesetters achieve good results, as one or two of the physicians I spoke with reason, it still does not justify endorsing their craft, since the bonesetters' training and practice are unstructured. The injured continue seeking bonesetters, so physicians find themselves having to moderate their strictures and look the other way. In the end, since few people bring their traumatic injuries to the health centers, as attested by data from the Comalapa and San Pedro La Laguna Health Centers, and since health center physicians by their own account have not been able to correct such injuries themselves, physicians permit the bonesetters to carry out a de facto practice.

As a result of this troubled conversation with biomedicine, Maya bonesetters have had to make adjustments to their work. In Comalapa, for instance, although bonesetters never advertise, bill themselves as popular physicians, or give analgesic injections, they have become more selective about the clients they accept. They seem more inclined to treat only those cases with which they have proven experience, with the result that in Comalapa today there are probably fewer bonesetters who accept fracture cases than there were thirty or forty years ago. This has meant that Comalapans have fewer traditional bonesetters to turn to and suggests that as local people notice bonesetters shrinking in number, they might be discouraged from bringing severe trauma cases to them. One can envision how, as fewer people are entrusted with fracture cases, fewer local curing vocations may develop, prompting the injured to seek help from under-experienced health workers or outside the town.

The situation is somewhat different in the lakeside communities. One bonesetter in San Pedro La Laguna, Lázaro, advertises his services by using a business card. He even reportedly injects some clients with an analgesic/NSAID, though he tries not to draw attention to this (and might be phasing out this practice). On the whole, though, bonesetting has remained comparatively visible in San Pedro La Laguna and San Juan la Laguna, something that seems to correlate with how lakeside bonesetters are generally more open to receiving more serious cases, including fractures, than are Comalapa bonesetters. This suggests that whether for reasons of community reputation, the broader skill set of local bonesetters, or other factors, residents of the lakeside towns have many bonesetters to turn to and to perhaps serve as an example for future bonesetters. But whether or not bonesetters or bonesetters-to-be are seeing their skill sets increase or remain the same in individual settings, they are undeniably working in environments with a growing Western presence. With the entry of biomedical resources into the countryside, highland Maya bonesetters have been faced with either rejecting or assimilating technological elements that have increasingly become part of the health landscape and that structurally challenge the manual basis of their work.

The Entry of Radiography

Radiography is becoming increasingly available in rural areas and is found in San Juan Comalapa, but not in the lakeside towns at the time of this research. Injured persons in San Pedro La Laguna and San Juan La Laguna who want to get X-rayed must take a boat or bus to the departmental capital, Sololá, where radiographic facilities are available. Even though Maya bonesetters rely on their hands to diagnose and treat injuries, and clients know this, many clients bring X-rays of their injuries to bonesetters in these towns. Many Maya people consider radiography to be potentially useful in the treatment of bodily injury and expect bonesetters to be familiar with it. But instead of seeing radiography as presaging the demise of bonesetting, we might consider how bonesetters are actually approaching the technology. I have found that bonesetters, by expanding the boundaries of their practices to include radiography or other biomedical elements, are preserving valued native techniques while adapting to a changing health milieu. This has enabled Maya bonesetters to continue working but has also placed them at a difficult crossroads. Their craft must now reconcile elements from different traditions in such a way that newer elements serve the healing process without eclipsing the craft itself.

The radiographic challenge to local practice is not new. When it first appeared on the world stage in the late nineteenth century, this technology defied entrenched notions of body opacity that spanned millennia. Ten years after its appearance, it even prompted an English surgeon to describe how his fellows had believed radiography spelled the end of bonesetting: "The discovery of x rays made many surgeons think that bone-setters were doomed to early extinction, but up to the present time (1906) there is no evidence that it has had any tangible influence in bringing about that desirable result" (Thomas 1906:1034). Although he conceded that X-rays had failed to eradicate the bonesetters he so detested (and though he voiced caution about relying on X-rays for certain injuries), this surgeon could have perhaps foreseen a later development, namely, the nearly unquestioned diagnostic power X-rays would eventually be attributed. In fact, the X-ray and its sister technologies eventually unraveled assumptions of body opacity so thoroughly that body-internal imaging later became a hallmark of allopathic medicine (Kevles 1997:2). As these technologies grew in prominence, they precipitated the end to body-centered ways of diagnosing and healing. Western practitioners felt this shift most strongly. And as the following section outlines, the rise of imaging also set the stage for dramatic shifts among non-Western practitioners such as Maya bonesetters.

The Ascendance of Imaging in Biomedicine and Its Validating Role in Research

After Wilhelm Roentgen delivered his unmistakable images of living bone to the world in 1896, the possibility of deep body imaging was no longer just theoretical. It became both possible and, with the advent of the

Spanish-American War and the First World War, necessary. Observers have since noted the growing reliance on technology in biomedicine (Kevles 1997). A critical component of this, Sarah Kember (1991:59) argues, has been the production of graphic methods that ensure the primacy of the "Image-Eye" in diagnosis—the visually driven medical mode whose rise was charted by Michel Foucault (1994). In the last hundred years the use of the X-ray, in particular, reaffirmed and strengthened the importance of the visual faculty in medicine (Mould 1993). X-rays became the forerunner of the image-generating revolution and defined the imaging market for at least three decades following their discovery. They were later partnered to still more complex technologies, including ultrasound, CT, MR, and PET, today in widespread use.

The medical promotion of roentgenology, or radiography, began shortly after Roentgen's discovery and became but the latest way for physicians to distance themselves from popular bonesetters. Physicians of late nineteenth-century Britain and the United States had already registered their opposition to "unorthodox" bonesetters on the grounds that these practitioners had no institutional training (Marsh 1911; Paget 1902; Romer 1915) and that they claimed to employ intuition in their work (Joy 1954; Sweet 1844). The English physician Frank Romer (1915:5, 21) particularly refuted the role of bodily intuition in healing and became an early advocate of the radiographic diagnosis of injuries. Bonesetters of the time had performed well without radiography (Elliott 1981:255), but Roentgen's discoveries were impressing ever wider circles of physicians, and these increasingly considered the radiograph essential for traumatology. Bernike Pasveer (1989) notes that while the credibility of X-rays was initially uneven among technicians and clinicians, as radiographic practice promoted a new visual vocabulary and stabilized image interpretation, it became more generalized. The emerging favorable view of roentgenology was also held by the US physician John Sweet, who, though coming from a large family of bonesetters, observed: "It is my belief that the reputation of the Sweet family for skill in setting bones was often deserved; but quite frequently the blind faith created by popular superstitions covered up many mistakes in the past which would be revealed by the x-ray today [early twentieth century]" (cited in Joy 1954:438).[4] As Waterman Sweet intimated, from the turn of the century onward, X-ray technology would become increasingly important for distinguishing the "legitimate" work of physicians from the efforts of "unqualified" practitioners claiming intuitive skills.

Since that time, radiography has become so central to traumatology and orthopedics that its absence from bonesetting traditions has been taken by the medical profession to signify bonesetting's illegitimacy. And where bonesetters profess having intuitive abilities, official refutation of them is still greater (S. Green 1999). It is curious to note that though the bonesetters' lack of formal training was once what physicians criticized most about them, today bonesetters are as likely to be criticized for not using X-rays, among other things. Their nonreliance on this technology is evidence enough to physicians that bonesetters have not the tools to diagnose, much less to treat. To this point, and echoing the sentiments of many physicians, a Nigerian orthopedist argues that "the traditional bonesetter usually does not properly reduce the fractures and dislocations because he cannot make use of X-ray technology" (Oguachuba 1986b:170), avowing the connection between healing ability and X-ray usage. The necessity of X-rays for diagnostic accuracy is likewise argued in a mid-century medical text on fractures, which states, "The radiograph proves the existence of a fracture" (Compere et al. 1959:9). X-rays have been granted the final word in fracture detection, even though this detection does not guarantee that medical users possess the skills to actually reduce fractures.

Since their establishment in Guatemala City's San Juan de Dios Hospital in 1907 (Flamenco 1915:57), radiographic facilities have also been considered by Guatemalan physicians as essential to traumatology. For example, when asked if he could treat fractures, the state Health Center physician of San Pedro La Laguna, Dr. Arana, told me that he could but that he would have to know first, via X-ray, what kind of fracture it was. He added, "If not, I'll stumble into empiricism." Since he sends help-seekers to the departmental capital, Sololá, for X-rays, he is unlikely ever to reduce fractures himself, and, in fact, in his twelve years of local service he has never treated fractures. In dreading an "empirical" approach to fracture treatment, he disparages the hand-based abilities of Maya bonesetters, not to mention their use of the *baq*.[5] The physician in Panajachel, Dr. Vélez, also dismisses the bonesetters' hand-based skills and instead argues that people with suspected fractures require not only an X-ray to get diagnosed but also the services of a traumatologist *and* an anesthesiologist, and for this they must go to Sololá or Guatemala City. Physicians in Comalapa have made similar statements about the central role that X-rays play in diagnosis (Hinojosa 2002:33). As recently as 2018, Dr. Sotz', of the Comalapa Health Center, reiterated that if a person arrives with a possible fracture, they straightway send the person out of town to get an X-ray. This means that people in an injured state will have to travel, at a minimum, twenty-eight kilometers to reach Chimaltenango or, farther yet, eighty-two kilometers to reach Guatemala City. Now, as in the nineteenth century, physicians regard the use of sophisticated diagnostic technology as absolutely essential to care and as the mark of the "qualified" practitioner.

The validating quality of X-rays is also present in an array of medical and scholarly studies of contemporary bonesetters interested in assessing their effectiveness. On the medical front, authors use radiographic imaging to gauge bonesetters' work among bonesetter clients who present themselves to hospital. The literature on Africa is especially abundant in this regard (Bickler and Sanno-Duanda 2000; Steinmetz 1982), with much work focusing on Nigeria (Oguachuba 1985, 1986a, 1986b; Onuminya et al. 2000; Onuminya et al. 1999; Oyebola 1980). Outside of Africa, medical examinations of bonesetters' work using X-rays appear less frequently, for example, in Taiwan (Huang 1986) and Nepal (Strowbridge and Ryan 1987). Meanwhile, there is limited scholarly literature on bonesetters who incorporate X-ray images (McMahon 1994), but other works do draw attention to bonesetters' use of radiographic images brought to them by some clients (Ariës et al. 2007; Hinojosa 2004b; Oths 2002) or radiographic images that the bonesetters themselves take (Attewell 2016).

Medical and scholarly writings use X-rays to buttress their arguments but raise different points about bonesetting. Medical writings use radiographic findings to support physicians' suspicions that traditional bonesetting results in fractural nonunion and can lead to other problems. Extreme cases are featured, sometimes involving limb gangrene and amputation (Bickler and Sanno-Duanda 2000; Garba and Deshi 1998; Onuminya et al. 1999; Onuminya et al. 2000; Strowbridge and Ryan 1987). Despite individual case outcomes, these works insist that bonesetters perform poorly and offer X-ray material as first-tier evidence of this. Medical writings caution physicians to be aware of local healers, including bonesetters, whose work they can expect to have to repair. The scholarly, ethnographic work of McMahon (1994), meanwhile, utilizes X-rays and arrives at another conclusion. Radiography confirms his experience of a bonesetter's successful work, and, to this effect, he provides "before bonesetter" and "after bonesetter" images of the injury. Even with these relatively few studies, we can see how X-rays can be used to support a variety of positions on bonesetters' work, with caution that the findings of these studies vary depending on the injuries researched and the person who bears them. Physicians typically see trauma cases that bonesetters could not resolve and that often present in advanced states of ossification or necrosis. Their exposure to bonesetters' work is, therefore, biased against successful bonesetter treatments. McMahon (1994), on the other hand, documents treatment by a bonesetter subsequent to poor treatment by a physician at a hospital, suggesting that, in this case as in the preceding, the best of the initial caregiver's efforts may not be reflected.

Significantly, the researchers use radiographs in similar ways. In each case the image is considered a source of objective and accurate data.[6] Its inclusion strengthens the author's conviction and is intended to dispel doubt in the reader. Perhaps it is not surprising, then, that this technology has become a critical marker of social authority when Western medicine confronts Maya bonesetting. As the bearer of the technological standard, biomedicine claims ownership not only of the visually compelling X-ray but also of authority over the body it commands. With this claim, biomedicine restricts the legitimate exercise of authority to those using the approved technology. In doing so, it refutes the place of bodily insight in healing, supplanting the hands with the radiograph. Whereas before, only Maya bonesetters and midwives could claim direct insight into bodies in Guatemala, now X-rays allow other individuals direct access to internal and structural bodily information in the visual format so dominant in biomedicine (Gordon 1988:32; Jay 1986), a format that is highly sophisticated and that allows for many possibilities of manipulation (Sierra Hernando 2014). In practical terms, technicians can generate a visible picture of what the bonesetters' hands sense. Imaging suggests an alternative to local forms of knowledge, which have rested on a tactile and embodied premise.

X-rays and Their Limitations

For two important reasons, bonesetters have not embraced X-rays in wholesale fashion. First, X-rays are associated with physicians and technicians who, bonesetters believe, have not performed well with musculoskeletal injuries. Second, they represent an added cost in terms of travel, lost wages, and direct expense for the injured person's family. Given how X-ray seeking entails additional efforts in the pursuit of uncertain benefits, bonesetters have not sought to broaden the use of the technology for the technology's sake alone.

Still, it is not unusual to see bonesetters looking over X-ray images while working on clients. Kaqchikel and Tz'utujiil bonesetters report that many clients visit them having already X-rayed their injuries. The Comalapan bonesetter Tomás says, "Yes, yes, yes, the majority arrive with their radiographs, they come with their radiograph and say, 'Here is your radio-graph.'" He clarifies, though, that "there are machines that don't detect [fractures] . . . [T]hat's where I come in and see if it's broken." Tomás cautions that while X-rays usually reveal fractures, he must have the final word on determining a fracture. The Comalapan Rómulo agrees that X-ray images have their limitations and adds that radiographic technicians do not really know about human bones and can mistakenly tell their clients that nothing is wrong with them. He feels that the specialist interpretation usually connected with the imaging is not to be trusted. For individuals such as Tomás and Rómulo, then, X-rays only moderately augment their hand-based knowledge and do not contribute directly to their therapeutics. As a technology appealing largely to the visual, radiography is of far less importance to Maya bonesetting than it is to Western medicine.

Popular misunderstandings of the X-ray have also, at times, discredited this instrument among Mayas. In Guatemala, technical knowledge of these devices is limited to a few technologists and radiologists, leaving the rest of the population with only a vague understanding of them at best. For Mayas, in particular, the nature of the rays is so mysterious that many attribute fracture-curing abilities to them. As part of their description of biomedical treatments, Mayas sometimes speak of how they went to a physician, got X-rayed, and still did not get cured, revealing that they think of X-raying as a curative procedure. Needless to say, to discover that X-rays are not curative likely disappoints Maya users, compounding their existing difficulties with biomedicine.[7]

To its detriment, X-ray usage creates delays and additional costs in treatment, not to mention misinterpretations of data. Even Western specialists admit that certain injuries, such as stress fractures, are not always detectable on X-ray film (Scheffer and Tobin 1997:334; see also Marlin 1932:61). But while Maya bonesetters are the first to say that radiography has its limits, they still have to engage with this technology and its new bearers. In the meantime, this technology is becoming yet one more factor affecting how referrals take place among an assortment of practitioners.

X-rays, Referrals, and Professional Asymmetry

Maya usage of biomedical technologies is conditioning the practice of outside referrals. Casting, like radiographic imaging, takes place in a context of multiple health resources, and the presence of these resources reminds one that different formal specialists can enter the chain of treatment.

Bonesetters—aware of specialists such as physicians, biolab technicians, pharmacists, and X-ray technicians—have sometimes referred clients to these persons. Referral to nonbonesetters has become, in fact, increasingly salient to Maya bonesetting practice. If clients are in great pain, the bonesetter will almost certainly send them to a pharmacist or physician for medication. They will also send the client somewhere else if she or he presents with life-threatening injuries. Referrals of this kind, then, are not new. What is evident today is that when a bonesetter directs his or her client to another person, that person is often someone who can take X-rays. Referral thus usually takes place with respect to two elements— pharmaceuticals and X-rays—that are outside the purview of bonesetters' work.

Bonesetters do not normally refer clients to one another, though, as I mentioned earlier. Referral typically occurs in a structurally upward direction: either to physicians or to persons the bonesetters consider to be professionally connected to physicians, for instance, X-ray technicians and pharmacists. While some clients recount having gone from one bonesetter to another, this is usually because the clients themselves decided to find another practitioner. Alternately, injured people sometimes bring their injuries to bonesetters only to be told that the injuries are beyond their abilities; clients may then look for other bonesetters with the needed skills (e.g., the ability to reduce fractures). Injured people can and do exercise choice in selecting bonesetters.

An implicit asymmetry is at work here, however, in that physicians will not normally, if ever, refer a patient to a Maya bonesetter. Comalapan and lake-area physicians would probably oppose such a referral even if they felt that bonesetters could help in certain cases. Physicians typically redirect clients only to persons whom they consider to be structurally equal to them (i.e., other physicians) or whom they consider to be valid adjuncts to their work, for example, radiographic or biolab technicians. By regarding bonesetters as interlopers in their professional jurisdiction, physicians justify excluding them from their field of colleagues and auxiliaries.

In contrast to bonesetters, who sometimes refer clients to people structurally above them, physicians refer clients only to their structural equals or near-equals. The bonesetter's kind of outside referral, however, can help legitimate his or her work in two ways: (1) by showing flexibility in the face of dire circumstances and (2) by referring cases that would have proven too difficult for him or her, thus improving the bonesetter's overall success rate and bolstering his or her prestige (see Kleinman and Sung 1979:9). By conforming with the public's expectation that physicians can handle certain cases better than they, bonesetters benefit through the selective referral of clients.

The health-care terrain comprises agents of unequal prestige and resources. Still, Maya bonesetters have found ways to include people and use technologies from outside their tradition. When it comes to X-rays, even if these are noncurative and not vital to their craft, they are nonetheless striking and pervasive enough for some bonesetters to incorporate them into their repertoire. As the following section illustrates, the manner in which bonesetters have done this speaks more to their pragmatism than to the effectiveness of biomedical tools.

Beyond Diagnosis: Radiography as Confirmation

Radiography has made itself felt in Maya bonesetting primarily through its confirmatory power. As succinctly expressed by Rómulo, of Comalapa, it can augment and support what bonesetters find through manual palpation:

> Many times . . . there are [clients] that come, and they really don't believe what you tell them, you know. So what I tell them is that, "if you don't believe me [about the diagnosis], go and get a radiograph done so that you can see how it is, how the, uh, bone is." And everyone who goes, goes and gets a radiograph . . . [J]ust as I'd told them the injury was, that's how it shows up [laughs]. You see? So that's why . . . the Lord has bestowed this upon me.

If the client is unsure about Rómulo's findings, then he will recommend that he or she get an X-ray either locally or in the department capital. The Comalapan Tomás likewise recommends to some clients that they X-ray their injuries. He and other bonesetters are expected to identify in the image what has been detected by the hands. By drawing attention to an area on the film corresponding to a body part manually diagnosed as injured, the bonesetter is in a position to confer meaning upon the film (especially if the injury has low visibility) and thus to reassure the client. Since most Mayas are aware that X-rays exist and that they show an image of bones, with moderate encouragement they may agree to get X-rayed. In fact, many injured Maya individuals often plan to get X-rayed, even if afterward they fully intend to see a bonesetter.

As does the adoption of some pharmaceuticals, the conditional incorporation of X-rays underscores the overall empirical character of Maya bonesetting. If a bonesetter sees an X-ray, then he knows that the image should reflect biostructural conditions that can be dealt with mechanically. He may or may not directly see the damage to the body in the image, but both he and the client know that the damage likely had biostructural causes and that there is tangible physical injury.

Bonesetters who receive or recommend X-rays are getting additional validation of their work by those who consider the rays to have diagnostic value, even if they know the bonesetter does not use these images to diagnose. Rómulo does claim, though, that he can sometimes look at a radiograph and see where the bone is injured. His occasional interpretation of an X-ray likely also strengthens his clients' confidence in him, though it is predicated on a technology only recently introduced to his work. The recent introduction of X-rays to bonesetters has not precluded their being used for validation purposes in San Pedro La Laguna, either, as Lázaro demonstrates.

Lázaro seems to use X-rays more than any other bonesetter in San Pedro La Laguna. At our first meeting, as we discuss the injuries he treats, he shows me X-ray films brought by a man severely injured in a car accident. The images show fractures of both femurs and humeri. He assures me, though, that he "fixed" the man. Two years later, he tells me about another client who was injured when his bicycle collided with a truck, and he produces more X-rays. One image shows a fractured left radius and ulna, while the other reveals a fractured lower right tibia and fibula. Lázaro then produces X-ray images of this client taken eleven months after he had started treating the leg. The leg fracture, albeit to a layperson's eyes, appeared greatly reduced, though the bones were not completely aligned. Lázaro, who places film after film in my hand, seems confident that the X-rays speak of his skills better than he can. He expresses even more confidence one day when I accompany him on rounds in neighboring Santiago Atitlán and he introduces me to the man featured in the second set of X-rays. The young man, whose case I describe in chapter 3, relates how the accident tore open his right knee and caused multiple fractures. He was taken to the National Hospital in Sololá, where he was stitched, was X-rayed, and had his arm and leg casted. But when physicians told him that they would have to amputate his right leg below the knee, he left and went to Lázaro, remaining under his care for months. He is now able to stand and walk, and he shows me the scarring on his right leg as well as the slight deformity remaining on his right shin and left forearm (see figs. 3.4 and 3.5).

Although it is tempting to conclude that Lázaro has accepted the diagnostic power of radiography, several features of his interaction with the client suggest otherwise. For one, Lázaro accepted the client as a "refugee" from the biomedical system that endorses the X-ray, pointing to his dim view of that system and its diagnostic technology. Understanding the client's pain, and having seen such cases before, Lázaro immediately removed the hospital casts. Even after being shown the radiographs, he applied the baq sacra to the wounded body and let it diagnose the injury. He then used the baq to reduce the fractures and applied his own immobilization devices. Last, throughout the treatment, Lázaro administered salves and had the man take an antirheumatic, an NSAID.

On the whole, Lázaro evinces a combined empirical/sacred approach to healing that accommodates a few biomedical elements. He makes incidental use of X-rays—initially when helping some clients validate the seriousness of their condition and later when showing them how their treatment has progressed. The latter measure is most reassuring to clients who have taken "before" images and who can now compare them with "after" images. Imaging specialists would dispute Lázaro's authority to interpret X-rays, but for Lázaro the bigger concern is how to treat the injury reported by the client, an injury that is revealed by the baq and, at best, only outlined by the radiograph. X-rays layer his working experiences with an intriguing but nonessential visual dimension and provide him with a biomedical referent for those clients who need it. This conditional use of visual tools is not unusual among bonesetters. Even bonesetters in India who value the visual dimension of embodied knowledge admit that visual tools such as X-rays do not tell the bonesetters everything they need to know about the body. As Attewell (2016:13) reports, even for Hyderabadi bonesetters who take and use X-ray images of their clients, "the visual cannot displace the haptic in the performance of reductions," reminding us that diagnostic images are useful only insofar as they can be used in concert with proven manual methods.

Rómulo, Lázaro, and other Maya practitioners are developing personally valid ways of understanding and utilizing radiography in otherwise non-Western systems. This should come as little surprise since people elsewhere have similarly responded with pragmatism and creativity when confronted with novel technologies. Marcel J. H. Ariës et al. (2007:569–570) have reported, for example, how some Ghanaian bonesetters not only study the X-rays that clients bring them but sometimes recommend that their clients take an X-ray to check the progress of the manual repair. On the basis of these images, clients decide whether or not to continue with the bonesetter. Similarly, a Bolivian bonesetter augments his tactile diagnoses with the X-rays that clients bring him, at times even ordering the images himself "to verify the diagnosis" (Salvador Hernández 2011: 125). Even in the United States people sometimes respond to technology in ways its makers never intended. Stephen Barley (1988:511, 520), for example, finds that CT scan operators construct understandings of the technology that are at variance with how the CT computational system works. Technicians perform certain tasks "ritually" when the CT malfunctions, reentering commands, rebooting, and downloading, even if these tasks do not work. They at times regard "the computer" in anthropomorphic terms. Hence, when problems occur, even persons trained (albeit insufficiently) to use a technology develop pragmatic, nonscientific ways of dealing with and talking about it. Given this, it seems understandable that Maya bonesetters who have no training in medical technologies would deal pragmatically with a new technology and incorporate it into their repertoire in nonscientific ways. Bonesetters develop personally valid understandings of X-ray technology within a framework of changing client needs and expectations, and they use these understandings to strengthen their healing effectiveness.

Even though X-ray technology arrived fairly recently in rural Guatemala, bonesetters are using it creatively to further their own low-tech healing work. The rays are also noticeably affecting how the bonesetters view themselves.

Emergent Biotechnological Idioms

Biomedicine's emphasis on the visual and technological occasionally surfaces when Maya bonesetters talk about their practice. Bonesetters sometimes frame discussion of their hands in biotechnological terms, even likening their hands' ability to know unseen tissues and structures to that of an X-ray. Consider how Rómulo explains his hands' abilities: "I don't use instruments; rather, one has simply to concentrate with the mind, and what I work with is, are, the tips of the fingers. These are, these are the best, as you might say; they are like X-rays when it comes to detecting [chuckle] . . . where the injury is. And thanks to God, you know, one locates those injuries and this is how we have also helped our fellow men." Rómulo states his position, interestingly, by first asserting that he does not use instruments and then by comparing his hands to X-rays in their ability to detect that which is hidden.

The importance that biomedicine places on the visual prompts other revealing comparisons between the bonesetters' hands and X-rays. Another curer, Lupito, of Comalapa, describes his hands in relation to X-rays, but differently than Rómulo. Lupito says of the injured body, "It's that it can be felt with the hand . . . [P]erhaps there are instruments to see, but since one is poor these can't be used." While he suggests that the hands operate in an X-ray-like sensory way, he also implies that the hands might be supplanted if the challenge they face is to be defined strictly visually.[8] Were this the case, then the X-ray, even though more expensive, could be preferred over the hands. Still, his comment speaks more to the pervasive medical emphasis on the visual than to any lack of confidence in his hands. But compared with his fellow bonesetters, Lupito does seem impressed with imaging technologies such as X-rays, noting that only trained persons can use them and that "today there are special apparatuses, they'll even photograph the veins."

These biotechnical correspondences are not new. Some fifty years ago Rodríguez Rouanet (1969) observed something similar in San Pedro La Laguna. When documenting how bonesetters used the baq on the body, he noted that "upon encountering the fractured part, 'the hueso' adhered to it as though it had a magnet. [The bonesetter] immediately proceeded to move the fractured bone back into place, at which point the 'hueso' (secreto) was released" (Rodríguez Rouanet 1969:63, my translation). The sacred object worked as a detective device, such as an X-ray, using unseen electromagnetic forces. This "magnetism" remains part of the lakeside bonesetter's framework for understanding the baq. For instance, the bonesetter Victorino said that the baq is "puro imán . . . porque ach'äp ri baq" (a real magnet because it grabs the bone). Similarly, as I mentioned in chapter 3, the bonesetter Imelda of San Juan La Laguna remarked of her hand-shaped baq that "the hueso is what searches for the bone . . . [T]he hueso is like a magnet." Even when San Pedro La Laguna bonesetters do not call the baq an electromagnetic device, one can see that they believe it to function like an X-ray. When I asked Flavio, of the same town, if clients ever brought him X-rays, he said no. But then, motioning as though he were using the baq on his arm, he implied that the baq probed the body like an X-ray is reputed to: "Just this tiny instrument, the hueso, finds where the fracture is." Nearly all bonesetters interviewed in San Pedro La Laguna and San Juan La Laguna use the baq's purported scanning and reparative abilities, much as Rodríguez Rouanet (1969) and, later, Paul (1976) described.

As bonesetters gravitate toward explaining their bodies' abilities in terms of X-rays and scanning technologies, an observation can be made. In ascribing something to themselves—how their hands work similarly to X-rays—bonesetters are also ascribing something to X-rays. First, X-rays require a lot of experience to be properly understood and still more to be effectively utilized. As I explain above, bonesetters often disagree with how physicians and technologists interpret the images and, in so doing, underline that simply having the images does not enable one to diagnose and heal. Second, like the hands, X-rays can be misused if the agent is motivated by profit and deception. This bespeaks how X-rays can be a boon to the informed, ethical user, but, like the gift that Maya healers often profess to have, they can also be abused.

The X-ray idiom is enriching the bonesetters' working vocabulary, and, as this happens, bonesetters are bringing the X-ray into their self-validation. By talking about X-rays, for example, bonesetters appear to their clients to be conversant with technology; by allowing their clients to seek and bring X-rays to them, bonesetters are permitting them to feel proactive about seeking treatment. And by likening the ability of their hands to the ability of X-rays, they appeal to their clients' fascination with technology. Referencing X-rays has even been useful to bonesetters when talking with researchers and physicians.

To effectively enable the bonesetters' self-validation, X-ray use must be recognized as a limited concession to the authority of biomedicine. For bonesetters to speak of *radiografías* and *rayos x* means that they acknowledge the powerful presence of biomedical institutions. It also underscores how biomedicine channels the dominant terminology and technology through Guatemala's dominant language, Spanish, through which the terms are known to Maya-speaking bonesetters. When bonesetters speak of X-rays, they often convey a sense of wonder at the technology, suggesting that it is far beyond their grasp. But they also convey their belief that the technology's images are not infallible and that they do not necessarily surpass their own bodies' diagnostic abilities.

As it turns out, the radiographic idiom has been useful to more than just highland Maya bonesetters. As a vehicle for "getting beneath the surface," radiography can generate powerful metaphors of discovery, even outside of health care. This is evident in Middle America, where a current of thought elevates X-rays to the status of a probe into not just the unseen but the unseeable. For example, during a 1996 meeting of Neurotics Anonymous in Comalapa (which I attended), the facilitators encouraged people to take a radiografía of themselves. They saw this as akin to a moral diagnostic that allowed people to probe their deeper issues. This scan could reveal not only physical structures but also intent and mores. In another instance, spiritists in Guatemala report using "invisible" X-rays (Cosminsky 1983:166), reminiscent of how, in the early days of the X-ray in the West, some people thought that these rays could see and capture ghostly emanations on film (Kevles 1997:119). The idiom echoes in the scholarly domain, as well, as Ricardo Falla (1971:98) refers to doing a radiografía of the Indian's mentality through examining his mythology.[9]

In these instances, X-rays purportedly make the invisible visible and, thereby, appreciable and malleable. Their ability to locate and isolate phenomena also prompts comparisons between the rays and the hands, and it places X-rays in the company of other medical technologies whose usage is concerned with both closing and preserving distances.

The Body in the Image

Radiography has become central to many biomedical applications. For bonesetters, however, while X-rays can be useful, they are not indispensable. Bonesetters comment that since physicians can neither diagnose nor properly treat with only their hands, they must rely on X-rays. Spotlighting this biomedical reliance on machines, Kember (1991:64) argues that "the empirical eye[,] which becomes detached within the medical imaging machine[,] serves as a metaphor for a lack which is internal but which has been externalized." With this she suggests that what sensory abilities physicians once had have been supplanted by the instrument's detection and recording capacities. This move from body-centered to image-centered diagnostics has also been noticed by the North American medical community. Speaking of clinical image-making, Jerome Kassirer (1992: 829) comments that physicians "are creating mental models of physical models, a process somewhat removed from the classical hands-on auscultation, percussion, and palpation." The previous diagnosing task of the body has become the task of the machine, and Maya bonesetters notice this.

The physician's use of the technology not only reveals the distance between clinician and object but also solidifies it. Even something so simple as a stethoscope formalizes and concretizes the distance between the two (Foucault in Kember 1991:55). This listening technology permits information to move in one direction only—the official direction—between discrete participants and in the terms set forth by official medicine. In similar terms, X-rays are intended to convey information only to official consumers, technologists, and physicians. They are not meant to convey information to incidental consumers, through whose bodies they pass to create an image. And they are certainly not meant to convey information to persons outside of medicine to whom they are shown (see Erikson 1996:4).

In Guatemala, the official encouragement of X-ray use reveals attempts at making an "objective" diagnosis and clinically isolating the medicalized site. This is especially evident in comments by physicians, who chide the hands-on, ironically "empirical" approach of Maya bonesetters. By appealing to a sense of medical objectivity, X-rays offer the promise of final accuracy, without the complications of conflicting medical opinions or nonmedical modalities. And although, as Christian Simon (1999) and Lisa Mitchell (2001) demonstrate, the interpretation of medical images can be quite nonobjective and socially charged, this is outweighed by the X-ray's promised objectivity and is actualized through a peculiar quality of the photograph. In Roland Barthes's (1982:196–198) view, the objective strength of a photograph is enabled by its apparent denotative status, its ostensible ability to be "read" without needing a code. While an X-ray is not, strictly speaking, a photograph, the argument applies: if what is viewed on the X-ray film is considered a radiochemical imprint directly indicative of reality, needing no codical translation, then its message is clear, its objectivity accepted.

Purported medical objectivity was likewise evident in the American promotion of chest X-rays for TB detection in the early twentieth century, wherein large numbers of lung images were systematically examined with the design of seeing predetermined signs of health and disease (Cartwright 1992; Pasveer 1989:374–375). In each case, what constitutes "objective" is standardized and assumes that body structures and pathogenic expression are consistent between bodies. Such determinations hinge, of course, on the ostensible fidelity of the image and its ability to frame what is otherwise invisible.

The official desire for medico-visual objectivity is also discernible in ultrasound fetal imaging in the West, by way of which fetal activity can be displayed on a detached monitor (Petchesky 1987) or, as Valerie Hartouni (1993:143) argues, by way of which instruments and relations inscribe and enforce meaning as they "construct peering." As used to allow pregnant women to "interact" with their in utero "babies" (Mitchell 2001) and reportedly "bond" with them (Taylor 1998), as well as to bolster abortion politics positioning (Hartouni 1993; Rapp 1997), ultrasonography has been increasingly implicated in the depiction of the body's medical, and even moral, "truth." It is promoted as a tool that makes biological reality available to authorized operators (Yoxen 1987) and, through them, to persons who accept the apparent unmediated quality of the technology. That ultrasonography is largely used upon women's bodies is telling since, as Susan Erikson (1996:3) and Ann Sætnan (1996:66) observe, it occurs in tandem with a structural discounting of women's knowledge. Further, when women's knowledge is expressed as midwife's intuition, it is deliberately challenged by the use of "technocratic tools of birth" such as ultrasound (Davis-Floyd and Davis 1997:319). Ultrasound practice enacts, and is enacted by, relationships of power while cloaking authoritative knowledge in medical objectivity. It hinges upon a validation and control of information that are also crucial to radiographic legitimacy.

X-ray imaging encourages the idea that injury can be isolated, captured, and studied at a remove from the sufferer. It promotes the idea that private, bodily information can be rendered visually, made public, and placed before a "qualified" interpreter (Cartwright 1992:23, 28). Within this scheme, the sufferer's descriptive abilities are discredited, subordinated to what can be seen and read in the image. If used as directed, X-ray imaging limits the sufferer's participation in healing by diminishing her or his ability to bring the causative circumstances of the injury into the diagnosis, something otherwise quite central to bonesetters' work. Even when X-rays are pitched as a tool of early disease detection and, thus, as something that individuals should seek, radiographic screening ensures that someone other than the patient (i.e., the physician) will retain final diagnostic authority.

Guatemalan physicians may hope that the perceived need for X-rays will bring injured persons within reach of formal health workers, whereafter they can be kept under their purview. But some Guatemalans are using the rays differently. Injured Mayas and Maya bonesetters are using X-rays to further participate in their healing without conferring wholesale authority upon biomedicine. The conferral of authority is conditional and not complete.

Radiography challenges the Maya bonesetters' legitimacy on two main fronts. First, with radiography, clients can arguably have their bone injuries diagnosed quickly and painlessly, which presents an advantage over the bonesetter, who is neither quick nor painless in his or her diagnosis. Second, radiography arguably renders less vital the ability of the bonesetters' hands to offer insights into the injured body during treatment. On both counts, the use of X-rays intimates that treatment modes such as those of Maya bonesetters weaken with the ascendance of Western technology. As something that graphically represents structural injury, radiography suggests an alternative to local forms of knowledge.

Although the bonesetter's manual modality and its underlying principles have been structurally targeted by radiography, radiography has not eclipsed the work of bonesetters in the studied communities. Judging from how bonesetters continue expressing confidence in their abilities, and from the way in which injured people bring X-rays to bonesetters when seeking diagnosis and treatment, X-ray usage has not undermined the patronage of bonesetters. It has not been the case that persons who receive X-rays thereafter seek treatment only from biomedical specialists, nor has it been the case that persons intending to get treatment from bonesetters avoid X-rays. Individuals and families seek radiographs for individual reasons and under individual circumstances, and sometimes they do so before deciding on a treatment course. There are indications, moreover, that radiographs are being reappraised by bonesetters and are being used to further legitimate their work. When clients are urged to get their injuries X-rayed, some bonesetters report, they are reassured about the bonesetters' abilities and even about their ostensible familiarity with this technology. Radiography permits the injured to feel they can participate in the diagnosis and make an informed choice about treatment. Observers of other popular health practices in Guatemala have long noted the ability of indigenous health specialists to engage with new technologies and sometimes incorporate them into their work (Cosminsky 1982, 2016; Cosminsky and Scrimshaw 1980). Many midwives, for example, have found biomedical elements—such as scissors, squeeze bulbs, and injections that speed delivery—useful albeit controversial adjuncts to practice (Goldman and Glei 2003; Hinojosa 2004a). For bonesetters, the limited admission of a novel medical technology into their work encourages a balanced engagement with clients and preserves their confidence, while it also preserves the state of relations between bonesetters and the technology's purveyors.

Maya bonesetters have opened an important place for Western elements in their practice, but this alone has not earned them the tolerance or respect of physicians. A practical and symbolic divide still exists between these classes of practitioners, one that will likely not be ameliorated by the bonesetters' selective adoption of biomedical elements. But while bonesetters have supplemented their empirical approach with Western elements, Western practitioners remain closed to elements of Maya healing.[10] This has added to the tension between physicians and bonesetters and, now as in the first post-Roentgen years, underscores the power wielded by medicine to designate legitimate and nonlegitimate knowledges and to enforce the boundaries between them.

Concomitant with their distance from physicians, Maya bonesetters retain their own ways of knowing. When a Maya bonesetter holds an X-ray film against the sky, he may be looking at an image previously seen by a physician. The film and the image may be the same, and the injury they refer to equally painful, but the act of viewing the image will mean for the bonesetter something quite different from what it will mean for the physician. Rather than considering the image a revealing shadow of the injury structure, the bonesetter considers it an obscure refraction of a body in pain. The image layers his embodied diagnostic experience with a supplemental vehicle of meaning, one useful for providing the injured person an additional frame of reference by which to make treatment decisions. Highland Maya bonesetters and their clients find this to be a useful quality of radiographic imaging and so allow its conditional presence in their work.

The wide acceptance of the X-ray throughout Guatemala that makes this folk usability possible also opens the way for another kind of radiographic operator, one positioned closer to the usual workspace of the bonesetter, the home. But as I explain in the next, closing chapter, this operator's work does not sit comfortably in either the world of bonesetting or that of biomedicine. Instead, his work reinforces many of the biomedical presuppositions about bonesetting we have seen thus far. It also signals some of the limits of cooperation between medicine and bonesetting that researchers and clinicians have tried to address in different parts of the world.

Conclusion. Defined Images, Hazy Roles: Scanning for Change

Walking uphill through Comalapa's Tz'an Juyu' neighborhood one morning, I eventually reach the home of someone who I heard runs an X-ray service out of his house. It is not the home business one usually hears about in Comalapa, so I want to see it for myself. When I knock on the door and ask for Felipe, the woman who answers the door, Felipe's wife, tells me he is not yet home but that I am welcome to come in and see the machine they use. Stepping into the main room of the house, I look to my left and see a seven-foot-high metal device standing on the floor, its extension arm affixed to an X-ray tube head. The head points downward to a narrow wooden utility table, almost directly at an electric clothing iron sitting below the head's aiming cylinder. On the wall by the door, where in other homes a calendar or school diploma might be displayed, hangs an X-ray film illuminator.

Mariana, Felipe's wife, tells me that the machine is actually a dental X-ray machine that Felipe bought in separate pieces in Chimaltenango and put together little by little. When Felipe arrives a short while later, he greets me and describes how the device was not working when he bought it secondhand from the friend of a dentist who had left for the United States, but that he eventually got it to work. And though it is a dental X-ray, he explains, "la misma necesidad hace que saque sus radiografías de hueso" (out of necessity it has to be used to take bone radiographs). That the machine takes these radiographs in a completely unshielded space is obvious to the eye, as is its positioning next to a wall adjoining a neighbor's house. Felipe assures me, though, that the machine and its use are completely safe. Mariana clearly agrees with him; she irons clothing on the scanning table when the device is switched off. They behold the machine today with the pride of a household that just bought a new car or

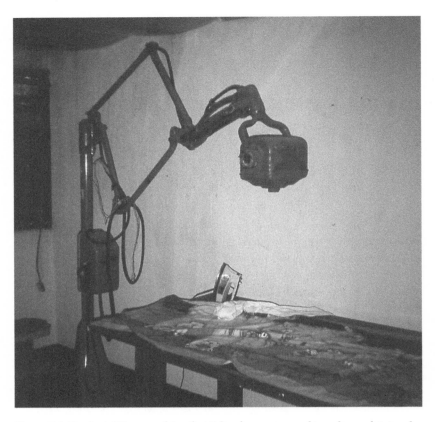

Figure 5.1. The dental X-ray machine that Felipe has repurposed to radiograph injured people in his Comalapa home. Note the family's electric iron propped on the utility table. Photo by Servando Z. Hinojosa.

new land, and it no doubt represents a big expense for them. Arriving at this point, however, has not been easy for Felipe, and his description of his work outlines a couple of the unexpected turns that brought him here. It also suggests that questions about where he fits among other people concerned with health, including bonesetters, may go unanswered for a while.

By Felipe's telling, his has been an accidental career. He had been working as a bricklayer, building a local private hospital, and when staffers there announced that they needed some workers to get trained as medical technicians, Felipe saw an opportunity. He put his name in the hat and was eventually chosen as one of three people to receive training as an X-ray technician at the privately funded Behrhorst Clinic in Chimaltenango. His training there lasted a year, and after he earned the certificate that now hangs on his wall, he was able to find work that paid about eighty quetzals a week. But this was not enough for his family to live on, so in a bid to acquire a state-issued certificate, and thus increase his earning potential, he began taking Saturday classes at the national Social Security Institute in Guatemala City for yet another year. With the additional radiographic training and diploma he received, he is now able to make much more money, up to four hundred quetzals a week. To make this amount, he has had to keep two jobs, one at the National Hospital in Chimaltenango and the other at a private clinic. Working at these two places has meant a lot of commuting, but it fits well with his income objectives. In fact, his drive for higher income takes pride of place as the main motivator in his work. The prospect of learning something new and investing time in it made sense to him only insofar as he earned the desired compensation. This does not mean that Felipe has not taken a keen interest in radiography. He knows it is an uncommon specialty, and the technological expertise he has gained along the way makes up a big part of how he sees himself. But these changes have not dissolved his ties to Tz'an Juyu', and he still tries to keep one foot in the neighborhood.

So deliberately does Felipe try to stay connected to his roots that he uses the neighborhood as a key reference point in his self-construction. At different points in our conversation he portrays himself as a man of the people, insisting that he is striving to make his services accessible to those who live nearby. He describes, for one thing, how little he charges. Whereas clinics in Chimaltenango will charge someone Q90 to Q125 for a single X-ray image, Felipe's service costs much less, as little as Q50, says Mariana. She adds that some people cannot afford even this, so they accept just Q20 from them. With these modest fees, Felipe says, "la gente queda agradecida" (people really appreciate it). They might charge people even less but for the need to purchase film, chemicals, and other supplies, as well as equipment. In the meantime they keep their lab setup very basic, using plastic buckets instead of elaborate film-developing trays.

Felipe also stresses his commitment to his neighbors when describing his interactions with physicians, especially in the context of a big business decision. He says that physicians in Chimaltenango have asked him to sell them his X-ray machine, but he refuses. He will not sell because the machine "es necesidad de la población . . . [A]l pueblo le hace falta" (it's a town need . . . [T]he people need it). But though his phrasing implies that he sides completely with the popular sector, other considerations are at work. As I discuss below, while many of his stated allegiances are to the people, his project of self-construction is unfolding in ways that reveal his overall support for establishment medicine, even if this support undermines some of its mandates. Felipe enacts a pragmatic flexibility regarding some key features of biomedicine like diagnosis and referral, but leaves unchallenged other of its positions, such as its views of bonesetters.

We see his support for biomedicine initially in his opinion that radiography should exercise an adjunct role in this field. For Felipe, radiography is "un apoyo a la medicina" (a support for medicine), along with other technologies like *tomografía* (CT) and *resonancia magnética* (MR). His sees his role as providing the right tools for others to diagnose with, and says that he does not do any diagnosing himself. But right after saying this, he goes on to detail how this is only partly true. When Felipe develops images for clients, he looks for signs of injury to bone. If he sees any, he points to the film and tells them, "Esto es lo que tiene" (This is what you have), followed by "toma su reposo, esto se sana" (take your rest, this gets better). In actuality, then, he does offer diagnoses in what seem to him more obvious or apparent cases. If the case is difficult, he calls the physician he works for in the private clinic in Chimaltenango and asks him: What should I do in this case, should I send them to you, should I send them to the hospital, should I send them to another physician? He will thus refer clients exclusively to biomedical specialists like this one, people with whom he identifies professionally. In his view, this is acting in patients' best interest and speaks to his knowledge of injury. Nonetheless, Felipe is not the kind of person most injured Guatemalans attribute knowledge about injury to or seek help from first. He may live and commute in the spaces where everyday people get injured, but he aligns himself with a world that harbors a dim view of Maya bonesetters, and his neighbors probably sense this. In fact, he does not conceal his disdain for bonesetters at all.

When I tell Felipe about the bonesetters I have been meeting, he immediately frowns. He explains that bonesetters seem to think that many conditions are *safaduras* (dislocations) when they are fractures. He says that dislocations occur only in the joints, explaining that if the pain is only in the middle of the bones, then it is a fracture. Felipe does not think bonesetters or other people understand this. He goes on to differentiate between what a bonesetter knows and science, insisting that "el huesero no tiene conocimiento anatómico . . . [E]s [nadamás] un don" (the bonesetter doesn't have knowledge of anatomy . . . [I]t's [just] a gift). For Felipe there is no uniformity of knowledge among bonesetters, either, reinforcing the sense that they do not go through a structured education, only an informal learning process. As a result, "ellos no tienen conocimiento exacto, unos más saben . . . pero hay otros que no" (they are not exact in

what they know, some know more . . . but there are some who don't). The
idea that some bonesetters know less than others speaks poorly of bonesetters, in general, according to Felipe. He points out, though, that physicians themselves vary a lot in their knowledge of bones. As he puts it, "No
todos los médicos conocen los huesos, tienen areas de especialidad. ¿Qué
va saber un ginecólogo de los huesos?" (Not all physicians know about
bones; they have different specializations. What would a gynecologist
know about bones?) Still, while he distinguishes bonesetters as a group
from physicians, and recognizes that physicians have distinct specialties,
he does not question the legitimacy of physicians or medical knowledge.
This judgment he reserves for bonesetters.

Listening to him, there seems little to distinguish his ways of speaking
from that of physicians. He sounds a lot like a physician when he talks
about bonesetters, just as when he talks about key markers of biomedicine. For example, he sees X-rays as unequivocal windows into the body,
lauding the image-making power of the machine. Felipe also takes pains
to emphasize his training and licensing and describes his resulting income
opportunities in great detail. He likewise makes referrals as biomedical
providers do, expressing a clear sense of the qualified practitioners. This
means that while a local bonesetter like Tomás can and does refer clients to
Felipe, Felipe will certainly not refer clients to him or to other Maya bonesetters. During his vocational self-construction, then, and even though he
takes an unorthodox approach to diagnosis, he has been unable to avoid
taking on biomedically driven views of bonesetters.

One might get the impression that Felipe's work would be favored by
most physicians, who, like Felipe, disparage bonesetters and lay claim not
just to the body but to authorized representations of the body (Sierra
Hernando 2014). But even though he talks in ways local physicians would
mostly agree with, and abides by the visual vocabulary dominant in biomedicine, his work still sits uncomfortably with physicians. For one thing,
he works out of his home and uses a personal machine. By working a machine outside of a clinical context, he is seen as overstepping the authority that even his radiographic technician certificate affords him. For
another, even though he has taken biomedical pathways of learning and
uses approved technology, he is providing diagnoses to clients, including
of severe injuries. So while the establishment may have conferred some
authority upon Felipe, this is only because he has been trained through
establishment channels and accepts physicians as the highest authority,
and not because the establishment recognizes any ultimate technological
and diagnostic mastery over the body on his part. Physicians do not con-

sider Felipe qualified to image body parts on his own, much less to diagnose injuries based on these images. He positions himself on one side of the physician/bonesetter divide and openly casts his lot with clinicians, but they still do not fully see Felipe as one of their own. As Dr. Sotz' of the Comalapa Health Center says of Felipe when asked whether there are any local radiographic service providers, "Hay un empírico; no es confiable" (There is an empirical [worker] here; [but] he isn't competent). We see in Felipe's case, then, someone who aspires to be a more formal member of the emergency care team, but who instead finds himself cast in a supporting role, providing products that he hopes will become part of someone's medical treatment plan, even if they are just as likely to be used to verify a bonesetter's diagnosis, as I discuss in chapter 4.

Still, because his expressed loyalties to clinicians align with the larger messaging purveyed by biomedicine, his uneasy positioning ultimately affects Maya bonesetting, too. His voice bears the imprimatur of biomedicine, at least to everyday Guatemalans, giving him a certain standing in the neighborhood. He may not be people's first choice for injury care, but he can openly charge people for services like physicians do. His standing also implies that his injury-detection method holds more authoritative weight than that of the bonesetters. For Felipe and the clinicians he identifies with, even if some bonesetters have manual skill, they are more trouble than they are worth. He believes that the seeking out of bonesetters by so many people mired in pain points more to the public's lack of awareness than it does to any ability on the part of the bonesetters. He sees no upside to these workers, but admits that local people do want them and use them. This regard for bonesetters, crosscut with notes of indignation and resignation, reveals Felipe's many qualms about bonesetters and rings symptomatic of how the health establishment would generally prefer not to think about them and that they remain completely out of sight.

Filling in the Silences: Revalidating Bonesetting in a Biomedical World

In a setting in which physicians and their supporters like Felipe make the loudest claims on the body, bonesetters are reminded that their views do not count for much, if anything. Their work remains ever more consigned to those private spaces about which clinicians seem to know very little and to which they have little access. The aspersions cast by people like Felipe, among other concerns, make bonesetters wary of health workers and keep them below the radar of health authorities. Felipe reminds bonesetters about what they do not like about health workers, even though his role is less common than that of physicians, and even if bonesetters do not normally come into direct contact with him. As a result, despite the participation of Maya bonesetters in an immense field of action, they show little interest in becoming more visible. This may be because they foresee no benefits accruing to their craft or their clients in an environment of increased publicity, or because they simply want to avoid confrontations with physicians and their associated technicians.

It remains less clear, though, why bonesetters have also been rendered nearly invisible in the pages of Mesoamerican ethnographies. Bonesetters have received far less coverage by anthropologists than have other Maya native health specialists, as I have described earlier. So while we see timely coverage of specialists like Maya midwives (Berry 2006; Cosminsky 2016), plant specialists (Berlin and Berlin 1996; Kunow 2003), and calendrical ritualists (Colby and Colby 1981; Deuss 2007), when anthropologists mention bonesetters, it is usually only in passing. What focused anthropological research on bonesetters exists is confined to a few works. Exactly why anthropologists have not directed as much ethnographic attention to bonesetters as to other health specialists remains an open question, but it may relate to the relatively nonritual and nonesoteric world of bonesetting. Compared with activities like midwifery and shamanism, which can entail initiatory experiences and revealed knowledge, bonesetting might seem rather empirical and, alas, quotidian. Bonesetting also hosts a vocabulary of assumptions, practices, and tools different from that found among midwives, shamans, and herbalists, and requires a different approach. Such is the outlier quality of Maya bonesetting that neither has the Guatemalan public health establishment taken an active interest in it, a somewhat surprising fact since this establishment has in the past used native health specialists as a means of bringing their programs into Maya homes (Hinojosa 2004a). To fill in the silences left by these omissions, then, I have focused on this understudied group whose practices mend Maya bodies and livelihoods in the many places in Guatemala where their work was first incubated.

Looking at Maya bonesetters as a *single* group, though, risks overlooking the many differences among Mayas who care for injured people. In this study I have tried to identify their commonalities as a class of caregivers while also exploring what makes bonesetters in a given place different from those in other places. Then, by reviewing the work of specific individuals, I have also tried to give a sense of the variation of practices possible among bonesetters within single communities. In this way it is possible to view the uniqueness of each bonesetter's approach as expressions of the general type of bonesetting each community is known for. In the process, we have seen that although common traditions undergird bonesetting in specific places, these traditions do not bind bonesetters there to a common identity. As mentioned earlier, bonesetters do not see themselves as a unified assembly of practitioners, as members of a community of equals. Many bonesetters push back against the idea, in fact, that all bonesetters practice equally well. Their tense positioning toward each other actually presages the troubled ways they relate to a broader circle of more widely recognized specialists: physicians. And by and large, bonesetters have found it difficult to relate to these specialists, something having a lot to do with how the physicians' influence extends far beyond their individual clinical spaces.

Bonesetters know that even though the public has more faith in them than in physicians for some things, they work on a very uneven playing field. Unlike physicians, they can be learned of only through word of mouth and they cannot enter into formal business arrangements with clients. For bonesetters to practice anywhere other than private homes and remote fields could also attract scrutiny from physicians. So even though physicians and bonesetters both come up in everyday people's care decisions, and even though they both want to alleviate suffering, their possibilities for interacting with each other are tenuous. They cannot interact easily, and certainly not as equals. Other than in anecdotal instances of physicians and bonesetters knowingly working on the same injured person, it is hard to make out what any common ground between them might look like. There are still sizeable obstacles to this. For their part, bonesetters disapprove of how physicians diagnose and handle fractures. Physicians, meanwhile, cannot abide many features of the bonesetters' work, especially how they practice without any formal training. Much of what we have seen so far, then, signals the limits of communication and cooperation between Maya bonesetters and formal health workers in Guatemala.

The possibilities for engagement are narrow mainly because their approaches to care are so dissimilar. Without a doubt, they operate with divergent sets of principles. One group places the stress on an awakened bodily ability, and the other on diagnostic technologies that refute the basis of this bodily ability. One group works when and where the injured need it, and the other restricts its treatments to fixed spaces and hours. One group welcomes whatever payment the client can offer, and the other charges according to a previously set schedule. Moreover, when they talk about each other, and they do talk about each other, members of each group always single out specific cases that members of the other group handled badly. In this way one gets the sense that much hinges on the competing reputations of bonesetters and physicians, and this in turn hinges on where they got their knowledge. But on this count, although bonesetters do not discredit everything connected to medical education and knowledge, medical professionals do dispute the role of the sacred in healing and negate the idea of hand-based intuition altogether, preferring to credit radiography as the gold standard in diagnosis. This has made radiography, a highly recognizable biomedical tool, a touchstone for discussions about the legitimacy of Maya bonesetting as well as about its long-term viability. This technology's appearance has raised questions about how it might sit atop the bonesetters' work and even affect their future.

As I discussed in chapter 4, not only have Maya bonesetters not been displaced by radiography; they have come to use it in select ways. They have found it useful when clients need convincing that the bonesetter's diagnosis is correct, as well as when a follow-up look at a repair is needed, foregrounding what Attewell (2016:10) calls the X-ray's "evidential power." Even though biomedical workers indirectly try dissuading bonesetters from setting bones, the bonesetters are co-opting elements of biomedicine they consider useful. The bonesetters strengthen the relevance of their craft vis-à-vis some symbols of modern medicine, carefully adapted and applied, and bring X-rays, casts, and pharmaceuticals into the picture when it makes sense to them. In this way Maya bonesetters are weighing the benefits of a pluralistic approach to manual medicine. And though the way some bonesetters allow for and might recommend that clients use Western elements such as X-rays and drugs might imply that bonesetters are conceding all diagnostic and curative authority to biomedicine, the bonesetters do not see it that way. For bonesetters, using different tools means less a compromise and more an accommodation of new elements to meet local expectation of care. They are willing to rework some of their tradition if it suits their purpose and benefits their clients.

Regional Need, Uneven Care: Cooperation and Its Limits

Despite the growing availability of biomedical technologies, bonesetters are not letting their work fade from view. They continue working in an environment wary of their craft and its underlying ideas, and their services remain in great demand. With their emphasis on the somatically engaged, low-technology treatment of injury, bonesetters' work may run counter to official healing modalities, but it lets bonesetters keep applying their knowing hands in the provision of culturally meaningful care. It also lets them serve others in a context where vulnerability to injury is particularly high.

The work Maya bonesetters do is all the more salient because the people they serve, being "predominantly indigenous, rural and poor," are of a background the WHO considers especially vulnerable to facing health-care challenges.[1] As economically disfavored people with strong ties to rural areas, Mayas in Guatemala live, work, and travel in spaces where carrying heavy loads, walking on slippery surfaces, and riding high-speed vehicles threaten them with injury on a daily basis. They too often find themselves in the crosshairs of physical risk, and even when they get treated for injuries, they are likely to afterward carry on with daily pain and limitations. In this sense their overall physical vulnerability reflects a susceptibility to pain experienced by people of low socioeconomic status elsewhere, and even by people living in less affluent areas within otherwise privileged settings. Mette Brekke et al. (2002:221) thus report that among people living in Oslo, Norway, "living in the less affluent area was associated with strong and widespread pain . . . [and] with high levels of physical disability." By noting a correlation between living in less affluent areas and more frequent use of analgesics, they also identify a predicament that many people with chronic pain suffer when other options fall beyond their reach. Other scholars have also underlined the connection between living in poorer areas and having poorer health. Michelle Urwin et al. (1998: 649), for example, point to a heightened prevalence of musculoskeletal symptoms, especially back pain and knee pain, among inhabitants of "socially deprived areas." They signal a vulnerability to musculoskeletal problems that C. K. Elliott et al. (2015) find to be common in low- and middle-income countries, in general. In these countries, where some 70 percent of the traumatic injuries people suffer are in the extremities (381), it is virtually assured that people's work lives will be affected when they get injured. A breadwinner finding himself or herself suddenly unable to lift, sort, or carry what he or she needs to, or to simply walk, can mean immediate limitations on his or her ability to earn money or meet the basic needs of the household. Knowing that the breadwinner's injuries can lead to economic hardship compels many injured people around the world to seek help from others. They do this even if their chosen help-providers do not meet with the approval of physicians—professionals who often act as local power brokers and whose own degree of influence often exceeds their actual availability.

In many parts of the world orthopedic physicians see themselves as the best, if not the only logical, choice for trauma care, and they correctly point to their field's advanced diagnostic tools (Ariës et al. 2007) and to their considerable surgical capabilities (Zirkle 2008). But well-staffed orthopedic facilities are not found everywhere. David Spiegel et al. (2008: 921) state that "the majority of those injured worldwide have no access to an orthopaedic surgeon, and this is not likely to change in the foreseeable future." Speaking directly to the Nigerian context, Kenneth Eze (2012:2323) similarly observes that "musculoskeletal injuries are common in developing countries, but access to high quality orthopedic care is not." In Spiegel et al.'s (2008:921) view, this lack of formal care should spur the larger "orthopaedic fraternity"—orthopedists and practitioners from related institutions—into action, prompting them to take the lead in reducing the burden of injury in low- and middle-income countries. Not surprisingly, this is the preferred course of action among clinicians and their auxiliaries. Recognizing the sizeable logistical challenges this would involve, the authors go on to say that "strategies for teaching and training must educate and empower other health professionals to care for musculoskeletal injuries, where appropriate" (Spiegel et al. 2008:921), effectively spelling out the need to get other community partners to help complement the physicians' services.

Reaching a similar conclusion about lacunae in medical service, Eze (2012:2323) agrees and goes a step further. He proposes that in Nigeria, "traditional bone setters (TBS) serve to fill the gap, [even though] the nature and quality of their treatment are largely understudied." With this statement, Eze (2012) raises concerns that many fellow physicians have voiced about reaching more injury sufferers in parts of the world where most injured people seek help from bonesetters before they seek help from physicians. For him, the bonesetter will have a central role to play in helping physicians reach their care goals, but this will not come easily. As he notes, not enough is known about the bonesetters' approach and to what degree their care is even compatible with that of physicians. But if his goal is to get bonesetters to cooperate with physicians, its success could depend heavily on whether other physicians agree with him. As it turns out, many do, especially in Africa.

One has only to look at what different clinicians and researchers say about TBS in different studies based in Nigeria. When presented with situations in which people routinely take their injuries to bonesetters first, researchers such as A. Dada et al. (2009:333) say, "A suggested solution will be the incorporation of the TBS into the healthcare system so that they could be better trained and controlled." L. O. A. Thanni (2000:223) agrees the traditional bonesetter can be "usefully organised to provide safe primary care orthopaedic service," a proposal echoed by B. E. Owumi et al. (2013:56), who remark that "it is expedient that the government, in collaboration with modern practitioners to [sic] organize trainings for the traditional bonesetters." In their respective regions, these clinicians and researchers tend to concur that "the establishment of a system of education for these TBS will have far-reaching effects in improving their practice," as Eze (2012:2327) stresses.

While these researchers agree in principle that bonesetters should be part of the overall plan to reduce the effects of traumatic injuries, they have yet to agree on what collaborations between bonesetters and clinicians should look like. Current proposals center on a general "improving" of bonesetters' techniques, with an emphasis on having bonesetters actively recognize their limits and refer out many of their cases. They generally align with the approach voiced by Elliott et al. (2015:387) for Sierra Leone, who state that "there are many possible interventions, some of which are easier to implement than others"; "interventions can take the form of training rural providers, be they traditional healers or [those] trained in Western medicine, to treat patients with the conditions they can, and to recognize patients with what types of conditions to send to tertiary centers." In accordance with this, the formal bonesetter training advocated above deliberately intends to curtail bonesetter involvement in treating the injured. As Owumi (2013:56) puts it, official training "will also assist in referrals to the modern practitioners when treatment cannot be guaranteed by the traditional bone setters." So while he implies that bonesetters will take charge of certain cases, one is left to wonder whether his use of the word "guaranteed" speaks more to the consignment of a small number of cases to physicians than to a more hurried outsourcing of care by bonesetters.

Even though physicians tend to concur that bonesetters should have a limited role in handling severe injuries, there is some flexibility on this score. After agreeing that bonesetters can be "usefully organised to provide safe primary care orthopaedic service," Thanni (2000:223) makes a specific recommendation about what bonesetters should be equipped to do. Like other physicians in Africa, he recommends that workshops be organized for bonesetters, "to educate them on the need to refer their

patients for modern care after providing first aid including limb splinting" (223). He thus explicitly describes not only how they can be trained
to know their limits but also how they can formalize their role at the front
line of injury and actively apply their skills to fractures.

Clinicians like him are especially keen to retool and "educate" bonesetters because they have seen many problems resulting from poor bonesetter care. Topping the list of these problems are cases of limb gangrene
requiring amputation, resulting from excessively tight splints being placed
on limbs with broken bones (Bickler and Sanno-Duanda 2000; Onuminya
et al. 1999). Precautions against using tourniquet-like fixation devices
are especially urgent because many sub-Saharan bonesetters use tightly
bound splints of bamboo or wood on arms and legs (Eshete 2005; Eze
2012; Garba and Deshi 1998). But this use of tight splintage has presented
opportunities to intervene in short-term trainings for bonesetters, in
which bonesetters are enjoined not to apply dangerously tight bindings.
Onuminya's (2006) findings in this respect are encouraging. He offered a
one-day course to a TBS in Nigeria, including instruction in the safe application of splints in tibial shaft fractures. This resulted in a decreased rate
of iatrogenic limb gangrene and fewer amputations in the group treated
by this bonesetter, suggesting that even abbreviated trainings can make
an immediate difference (Onuminya 2006:321). Along with these promising results, Onuminya also saw lower rates of "infection, non-union and
malunion" (322). Acceptable union increased overall with the bonesetter
who undertook the course. Similar results following short trainings were
also reported by Eshete (2005) in Ethiopia, where high gangrene risks
likewise called for intervention.

In light of these outcomes, Onuminya (2006:322) recommended that
"the TBS should be trained as a traditional orthopaedic attendant (TOA)
for effective primary fracture care in developing countries." He determined, like Thanni (2000), that it is ultimately possible and indeed necessary to train bonesetters to apply proper limb splinting. Clinicians like
these, who believe bonesetters should be trained, have reiterated what they
think these bonesetters ought to be doing and what roles they should be
exercising. They have been equally vocal, though, about what bonesetters
should *not* be doing, and here their views diverge. Babatunde Solagberu
(2005), for example, would strongly disagree with Onuminya (2006) and
Thanni (2000) about training bonesetters to splint limbs. He argues that
although "some reports advocate incorporation of the TBS practice into
medical care delivery[,] . . . [the] training of plaster room technicians is
a better alternative [in Nigeria]" (Solagberu 2005:108). And though he is

not the only person to suggest training bonesetters to make plaster casts (Onuminya 2006:320), by calling for this he is effectively suggesting that bonesetters are better suited for this because cast making presumably requires a low degree of skill. The irony is that by claiming that cast making is a better match for the bonesetters' skill set, physicians would be consigning bonesetters to making the very types of devices that bonesetters generally associate with bad medical care.

In their own ways, then, clinicians favor moving bonesetters into more adjunct or first-aid-oriented roles, ones that support the mission of orthodox practitioners. To the extent that African physicians can envision working with bonesetters, they might consider them as being potentially helpful only under certain conditions, insofar as bonesetters can be trained to do their work very differently, referring, for instance, many of their clients to orthopedic care centers and treating those they care for according to strict rules (Eze 2012:2323–2324; Thanni 2000:223). A regime of medical training and supervision could purportedly help bonesetters recognize that some problems that clients present to them are actually beyond the skill of the bonesetters to diagnose and treat, such as cases of osteoarthritis and multicystic bone tumors (Eze 2012:2326–2327). In this sense, even though physicians are conceding that their own brand of service has fallen short in many places in which bonesetters have the trust of the public, and that their own discussions about the future of care have to include bonesetters, they still try to command the upper ground when relating to bonesetters. They continue to confer only conditional authority upon them. Enlisting bonesetters in a limited partnership, or to put it more accurately, in an asymmetrical referral arrangement, would still represent a big step for orthopedists in the developing world: studies focused on improving trauma care in these places often fail to even mention the existence of bonesetters in any capacity (Zirkle 2008), or if they do, they refer to them using disparaging language.[2] It remains troubling that studies of orthopedic care in the developing world tend to leave out or vilify bonesetters, but this vilification is emblematic of how the medical establishment, including in Guatemala, has yet to reach a consensus about how to address bonesetters.

Widening the Circle: Considerations in Integrative Care

Physicians in Guatemala have a generally low opinion of bonesetters, but I am not aware of any concerted effort by these physicians to formally prohibit bonesetters from carrying out their activities and to limit them to new roles. In the rare event that the medical establishment there were to agree on and enforce a more limited scope of work for bonesetters, as it has tried to do with Kaqchikel Maya midwives (Chary et al. 2013), the matter would probably remain unsettled. When medical authorities have tried to limit Maya healers to certain practices in the past, there is little to suggest that the healers have completely accepted these limitations, or that they would unreservedly accept new limitations.[3] If bonesetters were to accept more attenuated areas of work, similar to what we see proposed in African case studies, physicians might still raise concerns about bonesetters overstepping their given tasks. This could create worries about intensifying levels of alienation against bonesetters, ones that could preclude any good-faith outreach efforts in the future.

But since Western medical resources now reach into virtually every area in which bonesetters have traditionally worked, Western health personnel will have to continue finding ways to improve their standing among local care-seekers. They will need to make their own system of care more relevant to people who usually go to bonesetters before they go to physicians. This should encourage a reevaluation of where local resources can fit into a more inclusive medical system, because as we can see in different African (Ariës et al. 2007; Eze 2012; Nyamongo 2004) and Asian (Narangoa and Altanjula 2006; Rasheed 1985; Unnikrishnan et al. 2010) settings, injured people have access to both traditional bonesetters and services such as X-rays, and they make frequent use of both. There would be a need, moreover, to overcome considerable medical biases against bonesetters, an admittedly difficult proposal in a region such as West Africa, where physicians have routinely taken an adversarial stance against bonesetters and where they might stand to gain professionally by opposing them, as Burford et al. (2007:368) imply.

An enlarged approach to (co-)managing injury and pain could also benefit from more options for self-treatment outside the clinical context, ones potentially involving bonesetters. Therapeutic self-massage, for instance, is currently being explored for use in ongoing treatments for the hand and knee (Atkins and Eichler 2013; Field et al. 2007). When coordinated with clinical care, self-massage could prove especially promising for supplying long-term treatment of the extremities, the body parts that suffer the most injuries in low- and middle-income countries (Elliott et al. 2015: 381). Self-massage may also form part of a suite of approaches needed to manage injury conditions and physical limitations in areas where no orthopedists work, as well as in places that orthopedists work but where their patients seldom return for follow-up care. The latter amounts to a sizeable care opportunity because, as Zirkle (2008) notes, orthopedists have a lot of trouble getting patients to return to them after an initial care visit.[4] In situations like these, in which patients do not typically revisit the medical caregiver after the first meeting, a sustainable client-delivered, and potentially bonesetter-assisted, therapeutic strategy becomes especially worth examining.

It is still unlikely that bonesetters will be systematically brought into the conversation about improving medical follow-up rates or about helping with follow-up care. With a few exceptions (Hemmilä 2005; Hemmilä et al. 2002; Räsänen et al. 2005), there seems to be little official interest in exploring more integrated roles for bonesetters in caring for the injured and physically impaired. This is true even when the evidence shows that using bonesetters is associated with tangible benefits—the need to take fewer analgesics, fewer sick leaves among people experiencing chronic neck pain, and so on (Zaproudina et al. 2007:436). And since incorporating massage into medical care has also been associated with reduced pharmacological use when treating acute or subacute low back pain (Qaseem et al. 2017), chronic tension headaches (Quinn et al. 2002), postoperative pain (Le Blanc-Louvry et al. 2002), and other conditions, there is yet more reason to explore manual therapies further.[5]

Like most medical personnel, though, physicians in Guatemala tend to show little interest in what bonesetters might bring to patient care. With few exceptions (Car et al. 2005), there is little to indicate that physicians and bonesetters have found common ground and little to show that they are even interested in starting a dialogue. In the absence of any meaningful overtures by those holding the upper hand—physicians—the possibilities for physician-bonesetter cooperation down the road increasingly weaken. Bonesetters continue being marginalized and derided by those biomedical actors most in need of their partnership, something that could further delay any possible strategic cooperation between them. Rural health could nonetheless benefit if physicians, as influential stakeholders in rural areas, were to recast their thinking about Maya bonesetters at least to the point of suspending judgment about them, in line with what Guatemalan physician Icú Perén (2007) has suggested about Maya healers in general. But as it now stands, physicians see a future for bonesetters and bonesetting quite different from what bonesetters themselves do.

Maya Bonesetting Tomorrow and Today: Glimpsing Its Futures

Are Maya bonesetters in Guatemala moving toward becoming simply providers of medical first aid? I am tempted to say that there is some evidence of this in Comalapa because many manual medicine workers there do not address fractures. On the other hand, there have probably always been bodyworkers who focus only on massages and not on fracture reduction. The picture is inconclusive, then, but physicians probably still envision a more portal-of-entry role for bonesetters, one in which bonesetters provide first aid, *primeros auxilios*, and referrals to clinicians. Further unsettling the picture is how physicians and bonesetters have very different understandings of primeros auxilios. For example, when the Comalapan Tomás says "Yo hago los primeros auxilios a la gente" (I provide first aid to people), he seems to imply that he treats injured people as a first responder and then sends them to a clinician. But for him, providing primeros auxilios means not only that he is the first one presented with the injury but also that he is usually the *only* one who will deal with that injury. Numerous other bonesetters probably share in this view.

How much will Maya bonesetters have to recalibrate their work if biomedicine increasingly pressures them to take on a conventionally understood first-aid role, of applying emergency stabilization and referring to clinicians? If Guatemalan physicians intensify their objections to bonesetters and try to delimit their work (however unlikely this might seem at the moment), it could mean sizeable changes to bonesetting and could imperil some signature aspects of the bonesetters' work. Bonesetters might conceal their practices more, further limiting their visibility and reducing the number of people they attend to. They might also find it necessary to phase out certain practices, for example, fracture reduction, that usually draw the heaviest criticism from clinicians. But making these adjustments to their work would affect more than just the bonesetters' availability and scope of practice. Taken together, they could gradually erode the idea that bonesetters have special insights and skills, something that would almost certainly weaken the public's confidence in them and thus the bonesetters' basis for validation. With the recasting of bonesetting as a referral-heavy first-aid endeavor, there would be little to ensure the continuation of Maya bonesetting as we know it today.

Relations between clinicians and bonesetters have not reached this point, though, as I discuss in chapter 3, and for the moment each group still keeps a certain distance from the other. Neither group has intruded decisively into the other's workspace. In the Kaqchikel and Tz'utujiil towns discussed in this book, this means that bonesetters have largely kept their diagnostic and therapeutic practices intact. They have continued palpating and treating people because these people's injured bodies keep summoning them to action. And despite the dismissive posture of clinicians toward bonesetters, and despite biomedicine's reliance on fairly advanced technologies, bonesetters act with the knowledge that they must manually work the body and apply force to it when needed. So long as the specter of injury keeps presenting itself, bonesetters do their utmost to address it, even when they have to inflict pain in the short run. The fact that clients accept this pain, it is worth pointing out, signals just how urgently they want the bonesetters' care. They know the care will hurt at first, but enlist the help anyway. That so many people prefer visiting bonesetters, even where there exist formal practitioners, also suggests that bonesetters have a different way of relating to the client's reported pain than do clinicians: Maya bonesetters accept and validate the sufferer's pain report akin to how folk massagers do this elsewhere (Hinojosa 2008:201–203).[6]

Bonesetters work with what clients tell them about their bodies, rather than with what scans or clinical tests tell them about the clients' bodies. But there is more. By acknowledging the sufferers' pain and caring for them, the bonesetter may be doing more than just restoring bodily integrity and mobility. He or she might be helping people move away from their identity as a victim of injury, helping them transition from a state of being unable to perform their normal duties to a state of being able to do so. Inability to perform "normal daily activities" makes up a big part of how Elois Berlin and Brent Berlin (1996:55) understand the state of being a "patient" among highland Mayas of Chiapas; it is not about simply feeling unwell but about being unable to do basic tasks. Mayas experiencing role interruption due to bodily injury need practitioners that can get them literally back on their feet and back into their workspaces, and bonesetters set out to help them with this in mind.[7] Limits do exist to helping people recover their abilities, though. And since the effects of injury can persist in the household for months or years, they remind us that in indigenous Guatemala the locus of injury, just as the locus of well-being, is the family. When an injury occurs, the problem goes well beyond the edges of the injured person's body. The future of that individual's entire family can hang in the balance, especially if the injured person is a breadwinner and is left unable to work because of the injury. Until the affected person finds the right manual caregiver, they might see little or no way forward.

Most bonesetters can empathize with someone in this position because they have been in this position. They have felt their backs stiffen following a car crash, their joints ache with arthritic rigidity, or their knees grind from years of carrying loads. Bonesetters feel bound to help, even if their way of helping does not resemble that of formally trained caregivers. Bonesetters want to help even if it means clinicians might notice them and speak badly about them. And yet, if they are worried about attracting unwanted attention, it really does not show. My impression is that bone-setters do not put much stock in what physicians say about bodily injury to begin with. They strain to accept physicians' credibility when it comes to treating traumatic injury, despite the elevated public authority other-wise accorded these professionals.

It is clear that bonesetters long ago put stock in a direct and hands-on approach to the body, one that contrasts greatly with that of clinicians (R. Anderson 1983). They do not see the body as simply a place to apply pharmaceuticals and radiation, as a mere canvas of pain that their hands can recompose or bind together on a whim. Nor do they see their clients as opportunities for personal enrichment. It would be more accurate to say that bonesetters regard sufferers first as their neighbors and kin, as people whose lived days are not so different from their own. After all, bonesetters spend most of their time doing the same work activities that their neigh-bors do. That bonesetters receive sufferers with a modest hesitation at first is telling, as it shows how bonesetters tend to play down their knowledge and do not actively look for new clients. What they do next, with a tactile familiarity born of years of handling, then connects to the real pains and limitations that people are feeling. The bonesetters place their hands on these suffering bodies, where an unspoken communication then guides their fingers. The transaction of senses that follows then moves through multiple channels, even summoning the curer's visual and auditory facul-ties. But while this interactive mode demands a very physical commitment from the bonesetter, the larger experience of bonesetting is not restricted to this; it is not defined solely by the bodily encounter between curer and client. The experience also grows from its encounter with larger structural realities in Guatemalan society.

The bonesetting practices I explore have been deeply affected by the diagnostic and treatment methods that institutional medical actors use and by the technologies underwriting them. Methods and motivations for Maya bonesetting come from within Maya experience, but because so much of today's Maya experience bears the imprint of biomedicine and urban life, bonesetting understandably reflects these, too. Much of Maya bonesetting has been inexorably shaped by its exposure to medical and Western ideas, institutions, and tools, making it necessary to take a wider view of bonesetting. It is worth considering that because of the weight of biomedical authority pressing upon bonesetting and felt by bonesetters, much of Maya bonesetting has been driven by an effort to distinguish itself from biomedicine. We see this especially when it comes to key markers of biomedicine: casts, radiography, and, to some extent, drugs. Bonesetters are selectively appraising these technologies, carefully adopting them at times and emphatically rejecting them at others.

While it is the case, then, that bonesetting has absorbed some elements from the larger medical and commercial world, it has also tried to present itself as standing, if not opposed to this world, in wary contraposition to it, at times more successfully than others. In a way Maya bonesetting must do this because if it fails to individuate or distance itself from the dominant health system, in the long run Mayas might weaken their confidence in it. They might see fewer differences of caring and skill between clinicians and bonesetters. If the perceived distance between them shrinks, and bonesetters either become harder to distinguish from clinicians or become increasingly dominated by them, it could create a real credibility problem for bonesetting. Bonesetting's future would be imperiled more by this than by the arrival of any one technology.

For all their vulnerability to institutional forces, Maya bonesetters do not sit around worrying about the long shadow of biomedicine. They simply lack the time. While some bonesetters do see fewer clients than others, all bonesetters also have their homes and their fields to keep them busy when they are not treating people, resulting in scarce free time. The demands of family life thus bracket their daily interactions with care-seekers, continually reminding bonesetters that every family needs for its members to be in the best shape possible, earn a living, and perform their household duties. This reality no doubt affects how bonesetters see an individual's suffering not just as an isolated experience but as the immediate sign of something else. Their clients' suffering speaks of group lives interrupted, of collective futures held hostage to pain. Bonesetters' living in the same precarious spaces as those they treat leads them to understand how a family's breadwinner one day can suddenly become the center of that family's season of troubles the next. Many people who approach a Maya bonesetter for care are shouldering this predicament, and whether the bonesetter they choose uses only his or her hands or pairs these with sacred tools, the treatment will work toward getting sufferers back in control of their lives.

At least, this is what bonesetters want, and what they try to offer as long as their own bodies allow them. Old age, and usually infirmity, takes bonesetters from their communities, and their neighbors feel the loss for years. But this does not worry Javier, who is still awakening to his curing skills in San Pedro La Laguna. Reflecting on his late father, the bonesetter Victorino, Javier tells me, "Se muere uno, hay otro" (One dies, there's another). I sense he is happy to be safeguarding his father's work, even if he keeps this to himself. We cannot speak for long today, though, because the afternoon is waning and Javier has many more things to do now than when his father was still alive. He takes up his shoulder bag and sets off down the dusty street. Somewhere a family is deciding whether they should carry their injured son-in-law to Javier or to another bonesetter, or maybe to someone with more years of experience under his belt. This is a big decision to make, but the family can rest assured that tracking down a bonesetter will not be hard. In towns and villages throughout the highlands, night finds bonesetters practicing with quiet forbearance.

Traditional Medicine and Bonesetting: Integration and Lessons

Calls for respecting traditional medicine have been gathering strength in many settings,[1] and many of these have fueled discussions about enlarging the current roles of traditional healers, even about integrating them into different health systems. Much of this conversation has centered on how clinicians and traditional medical practitioners might work together (Elliott et al. 2015), on how their respective resources can complement each other (Zank and Hanazaki 2017), or on how they might simply begin talking with each other (Anderson 2000:92; van Soeren and Aragon 2015:61). And while each of these lines of inquiry is relevant to distinct forms of traditional medicine, the experiences of specific kinds of healers in their encounter with clinicians will probably be different from each other. For instance, the interaction between a midwife and a clinician will probably strongly contrast with that between a shaman and a clinician. This does not mean that we cannot tentatively envision how folk practitioners might interact with clinicians, or even form part of an integrative care whole, but it does suggest the need to be specific when referring to folk practitioners. It might then be possible to see their potential for integration with biomedicine and, in the process, shed light on other lessons that traditional medicine can offer biomedicine.

Since this study focuses on bonesetters, I would here address how these two concerns—the issue of integration and that of important lessons—play out specifically to bonesetter experience. As I discuss in the two sections that follow, (a) the possibilities for bonesetter integration into formal health systems are uneven but promising, and (b) the most important lesson bonesetting may be offering to biomedicine is to focus on injury as an experience of the group, not just of the individual.

The Uneven Integration of Traditional Bonesetters

It is instructive to review the experience of a few societies when considering whether bonesetters can be integrated into formal health systems. Taking Bolivia and Hong Kong as a starting point, we see that while bonesetters get some official recognition in both places, the bonesetters' formal experiences are distinct in each setting. In Bolivia bonesetters can be examined and registered as a "specialty healer" under the auspices of a large government organization (Sikkink 2010:140). This enables them to advertise, charge clients, and operate openly as businesspeople with a market stall or storefront if they so choose. In Hong Kong, meanwhile, the integration of bonesetters with the formal health system has reached yet another level. There, bonesetters can be registered or listed according to the local Chinese government accreditation system.[2] This allows them not only to advertise, receive patients, and be paid for services but also to be reimbursed by health insurance and travel insurance plans. Many insurance providers in Hong Kong routinely cover Chinese bonesetting services (as well as acupuncture treatment). They offer to pay for bonesetting treatments, up to specified plan limits, by listed or registered bonesetters, as the websites of many companies attest. Bonesetters have here become closely integrated into the formal health system. Their use is so widespread, in fact, that at least one insurance provider covers treatments for injuries attributed *to* bonesetters.

Bonesetters in other places have not reached this level of integration with formal health systems, but indications suggest that local government and medical entities may be interested in this collaboration. For example, in Finland, the Kaustinen Folk Medicine Centre has carried out active research into the therapeutic effects of bonesetting. This facility has spearheaded research interventions comparing treatment outcomes of traditional bonesetters with those of formal practitioners in the treatment of lower back pain and neck pain, conditions that affect many people (Hemmilä 2002, 2005; Hemmilä et al. 2002). The biomedical gaze appears to be slowly enveloping bonesetting in Finland, even though neither the national health system (Social Insurance Institution) nor private insurance companies currently cover bonesetting there.[3] Coverage for bonesetting services is also lacking in nearby Denmark and Iceland, where official interest in bonesetting has not reached the degree that it has in Finland and where there is less evidence that traditional medicine is moving in the direction of licensing bonesetters and creating integrative care centers (R. Anderson 2000, 2004).

Nor in Guatemala do we see an official acceptance of traditional bonesetters. There has instead been a general call to broaden public understandings of health to include Maya understandings of health (Icú Perén 2007). Within this framework, a leading community health organization has looked favorably on the role Maya bonesetters play in areas where official health centers cannot fully serve people suffering from musculoskeletal problems (Car et al. 2005). The Asociación de Servicios Comunitarios de Salud (ASECSA) notes that in such places, Maya bonesetters may be filling an important gap in service, in effect revealing some of the limitations of rural health centers. The association and other community partners think that by encouraging the larger Guatemalan society to be open to traditional medicine, or to at least suspend judgment about it, some of its benefits can become better known and can better complement existing services. This approach, intended to value native health traditions, later comes to inform a WHO-driven initiative to uphold a general *derecho a la salud* (right to health) in Guatemala, especially of the rural and indigenous population, the country's most vulnerable sectors.[4] And as those people most prone to accident and injury (Peden et al. 2004:46),[5] members of the rural and indigenous population have often called on the Maya bonesetters' skill set.

While none of this means that Guatemala will be registering and listing bonesetters anytime soon, or at all, it does encourage the sense that the public can benefit from acknowledging bonesetters and other traditional practitioners in a way akin to the public's knowledge about and acknowledgment of midwives. After all, each kind of practitioner acts in accord with people's lived realities. But fostering a more formal acceptance of bonesetters will require more than simply accepting that they are out there and that they work. It may require some visibility of the kind that the Guatemalan government has in recent decades given to midwives and that it has just recently tried to bestow on another type of healer. A leading daily reported recently that the minister of health wanted to allow some curers to treat *mal de ojo*, a folk ailment brought upon by the gaze of another, in some designated health centers (Pitán 2016). If the plan worked as intended, and it was never explained in detail, it might have constituted a step toward the licensing of folk practitioners other than midwives. It would appear, though, that this proposal was made only after formal health planners realized that they were not meeting all the health needs of their constituents; theoretically, then, these planners might also envision a scenario in which bonesetters could step into the formal health picture in some capacity.

The integration of Maya bonesetters into the health system is untenable at the moment, but Guatemala has already accredited one group of healers and is considering accrediting another. This recognition, together with the fact that some local health workers are realizing the importance of bonesetters, suggests that health planners will have to take more notice of bonesetters in the future. Whether these planners eventually take a favorable view of Maya bonesetters may depend heavily on how Guatemalan society as a whole views indigenous culture. We have seen that with the more inclusive climate of interaction unfolding in the 1990s and the early 2000s, during what many called the Pan-Maya movement, Guatemalan society has shown more openness than before to recognizing the languages and cultures of indigenous Guatemalans. To the extent that non-Maya Guatemalans may also be valorizing some Maya understandings of health, this might also be partly attributable to the movement itself occurring against a backdrop of increased global attention to the lives of indigenous people.[6] This is a promising development not only because the Pan-Maya movement's call to respect Maya ways of being is reaching key actors in the country's education and health sectors (even if actions taken in response to the call have been uneven), but because this call might yet reach Guatemalan decision-makers in other sectors.

Also promising is the prospect that elsewhere in the world, some physicians may be heeding a similar call to expand Western assumptions about health to include recognizing the knowledge base in native communities. They may be broadening their definition of orthopedics, for example, to include traditional bonesetters as tentative community adjuncts who can size up people's injuries and refer more serious injury cases to hospitals. This is the case in Nigeria, in particular, but also in other African countries with large numbers of traditional bonesetters (Dada et al. 2009; Eze 2012). Some physicians in Ethiopia and Nigeria have also shown great interest in training bonesetters to diagnose and even set certain kinds of fractures and to refer other injuries to area physicians (Eshete 2005; Onuminya 2006), as I discuss in the conclusion. It is important to bear in mind, though, that while on the one hand, the physicians' outreach to bonesetters signals a somewhat more inclusive outlook on caregiving, on the other hand, this interest by physicians also entails marked attempts to scrutinize traditional bonesetters more intensely. The exercise of medical power forms a critical backdrop to discussions of compatibility between physicians and bonesetters.

So, without diminishing the value of collaborative efforts, we should keep in mind that the integration of traditional healers with health systems may in the end hinge upon both the disposition of the healers themselves and the type of health system operating around them. What the traditional practitioners want also matters. When confronting a powerful medical and economic system, for instance, some healers may even decide to curtail some of their services. As early as 1974, David Landy commented that in the face of dominant medical systems some traditional healers might accept their shrinking roles in curing, as he saw among the Tuscarora (1974:113). He also contended, though, that interested persons might also carve out a new niche in the emerging medical order, as Margaret Mead (1961:264–265) reported for New Guinea Manus healers who used elements of modern medicine to set up their own practices and even their own "hospitals." It may be in this light that we can understand Richard Anderson's (2004:14) description of how alternative-medicine practitioners sometimes emulate select elements of biomedicine. When biomedicine is ascendant, some healers might take up certain overtly biomedical practices or representations to compare themselves favorably with medical practitioners and even to show some of their own aspirations. These actions may have the intended effect of affirming the healer's knowledge or of providing visual referents for those of the healer's clients who favor visual referents, as we see with one Maya bonesetter who displays an anatomical chart in his workspace and with others who review X-rays that clients bring them. The selective adoption of biomedical elements reflects a fluid process of appraising and repurposing new tools in a pragmatic dialogue with practitioners' changing surroundings. And nowhere do we see bonesetters pursuing such a novel and biomedically imprinted course of action than in a recent case reported from India.

As Attewell (2016) discusses in his study from Hyderabad, a family of bonesetters has made a name for itself by redrawing the conventional technological boundaries around bonesetting. Not only do practicing bonesetters of this family use a personal X-ray machine to scan injured clients, but they routinely document their clients' treatments with these images as well as with other types of images coming from outside their clinics. One of these bonesetters has over time amassed an "archive of scans" (Attewell 2016:10), which he uses to review his clients' cases and, more important, to support his diagnostic and therapeutic authority. And because this family places a premium on its relationships with local orthopedic surgeons, one bonesetter uses his many images and scans to coax endorsements from these physicians. In this way he has come to rely heavily on, and increasingly define his authority in terms of, visual representations and the technologies that underlie them. In view of this heightened receptivity to new technologies, it might be possible to appreciate how amenable many Maya bonesetters have become, in their own way, to radiographic imaging. Like other Maya traditional healers (e.g., midwives), bonesetters have had to avail themselves of new resources and adapt themselves to the material inventory of an increasingly influential health system. Whether Maya traditional healers adopt new tools out of official necessity, because their clients use the tools, or because they personally like the tools, the tools are here to stay. It has yet to be seen, though, how much Maya bonesetters will change over the long term because of the new tools, or whether they will (continue to) adapt the tools to suit their craft. Neither is it clear whether their use of new tools will move bonesetting into broader usage.

These realities—the registration of bonesetters, insurance reimbursement for bonesetting services, how society and biomedicine value traditional medicine, and bonesetters' openness to new technology—affect the prospects for integrating bonesetters into formal health systems. The full integration of bonesetting into health systems is not preordained; the attention bonesetting receives in individual settings will affect whether bonesetters' work becomes formalized in those places. If there is high public demand for traditional bonesetters, for example, this could bring bonesetting into, if not the formal health system, at least more conversations about community health. A lot of the decision making will continue to depend, though, on formal stakeholders such as physicians. As they are actors with the weight of the health establishment backing them, any judgments about the compatibility of formal health care with bonesetting remain in their hands.

Family as the Locus of Treatment

Discussions about traditional medicine would also do well to explore whether traditional medicine can offer any immediate deliverables to biomedicine. One deliverable warrants special emphasis: the family, not the individual, should be the locus of treatment. Prior to discussing this issue, though, I will first note how biomedical practitioners reportedly approach the sick or injured body and then show how different this is from the way bonesetters work.

In their attempt to focus in on a body part or system, physicians have been said to decontextualize and even dehumanize individual bodies (Erickson 2008:100). Physicians tend to limit their clinical attention to observable signs in one discrete physical body, an approach that on the one hand allows them to access a range of classifiable data, but on the other separates that body from its familial and social context. Reducing the clinical examination to a strictly data-gathering event, moreover, fetters the diagnostic process and, as Carlton T. Mitchell (1989:48) argues, "leads the physicians to focus on the patient as an isolated individual." Given how Maya bonesetters also pay close attention to physically observable signs when diagnosing their clients, one might conclude that bonesetters' outlook toward the body is similar to that of physicians', that they treat the client as a body removed from its family context. If we think of bonesetters mainly as people who treat bodily limbs and tissues using a strictly physical approach, we might indeed be tempted to frame them as practitioners who are uninterested in their clients' daily lives and larger lived experience. But here we must be careful.

To think about Maya caregivers and their caregiving in this way would be to overlook an important distinction between physicians and bonesetters. It is vital to bear in mind that bonesetters do not treat the client as just a body part, even though they may be treating, at first glance, just a body part. As individuals who work and move in the same spaces as their clients, Maya bonesetters know that everything they do for their client will affect how that person will function as a member of his or her household. They know that every action they take will move the sufferer's family either a step closer to physical recovery and economic stability or one closer to debility and economic strain. Every move and every counsel they give will affect the family's ability to thrive, or just survive. Bonesetters are reminded of this responsibility every time injured people show up at their door, because injured people nearly always arrive with family members. The way family members support or carry their injured relative to the bonesetter points to how they all bear the injury, in a way.

That the entire family shoulders the injury is also clear in the way the family members take an active role in then describing the causative circumstances of the injury to the bonesetter. Together with the sufferer, the relatives co-construct the injury narrative in a manner similar to what T. S. Harvey (2008:579) sees among K'iche' Maya wellness-seekers in a healing setting. He reports that the companions of the wellness-seeker "co-narrate" the sickness experience (596). In fact, for him the role of the K'iche' Maya *yawab'* (sick person) is "inhabitable by multiple individuals" (583). They talk about sickness together because the sickness condition affects all of them.

The people Maya bonesetters treat also seek care with a "collectivist approach . . . to therapy management and decision making about patient care," of the kind that Erickson (2008:105) identifies in non-Western cultures. In a very real way, then, members of the injured person's extended family bear the strain of the injury, since they all feel the impact of it; everyone feels it, so they each have a stake in reporting it. This joint framing of the injury narrative, though, might not sit well with clinicians accustomed to identifying only one voice authorized to speak about a given injury event. But being open to this feature of Maya wellness-seeking can help the clinician access far more information about the case than she or he otherwise might and at the same time better gauge the case's economic seriousness.

Listening to the group's experience is one way for clinicians to grasp that sickness or injury is not an event isolated to one body. Sickness and injury conditions distribute themselves across a group of interlocking lives and create reverberations that can be felt for generations. For this reason, keeping the family as the locus of diagnosis and treatment may be one of the most important takeaways traditional medicine can offer to Western medicine.

Notes

Preface and Acknowledgments

1. I have deliberately chosen to use "clients" rather than "patients" because this kind of actor has a certain set of meanings in health-care-seeking settings. "Patients" implies a certain passive care-seeking, in my understanding, as well as a structural asymmetry between care-seeker and caregiver quite common in the West. I use the term "clients" because I am trying to convey that these health-seekers have more agency, they select among caregivers, they can refuse to follow up with care instructions, and they can go see someone else if they choose.

Introduction

1. In this sense, see works by Cosminsky (1972), Douglas (1969), Fabrega and Silver (1973), Gann (1918), Holland (1962, 1963), Instituto Indigenista Nacional (1969, 1978), Kunow (2003), Orellana (1987), Redfield and Villa Rojas (1962), Rodríguez Rouanet (1969), Tedlock (1992), and Wisdom (1940). I am also aware of one feature article on Maya bonesetters published in a Guatemalan newspaper for a popular readership (Martínez 2007).

2. Aside from ethnohistorical sources centered on Mexican Nahuas, bonesetters are mentioned in works by Lipp (1991), Odena (1982), and Sandstrom (1991).

3. Physicians who research African bonesetters tend to be very critical of them. Their publications typically report the failings of bonesetters and couple their criticisms with a call to properly "train" bonesetters (Eze 2012; Owumi et al. 2013; Steinmetz 1982) so that they might identify serious injury cases and refer their clients to physicians (Thanni 2000). Key among physicians' criticisms is the use of tight tourniquets by some bonesetters, which has been linked to posttreatment complications, leading to limb gangrene and the need for amputation (Bickler and Sanno-Duanda 2000; Brume and Ijagha 1985; Ofiaeli 1991; Onuminya et al. 1999; Onuminya et al. 2000). Researchers and physicians also express frustration that many fracture patients who seek care in hospitals often leave and seek care from a bonesetter (Solagberu 2005; Tijssen 1979).

4. In Asia, many researchers have published on Chinese bonesetting, and these works are unique for two reasons. First, they are often directed at orthopedic specialists who critically evaluate (Huang 1986), and sometimes incorporate (Fang et al. 1996; Shang et al. 1987), manual bonesetting techniques. And, second, they are also directed at formally trained bonesetters operating in an environment heavily affected by both biomedicine and Traditional Chinese Medicine (Minor et al. 2004: 93). Chinese reports often reflect methods (Li-Ming et al. 2016; Wang 2008) and materials (Lee and Lam 2001) used by bonesetters. In India, meanwhile, works on bonesetting often feature the continuation of bonesetting traditions, often in families (Nandakumar and Ghosh 2000; Panda and Rout 2011); their operation in highly stratified societies (Lambert 1995; Unnikrishnan et al. 2010); and their ostensible shortcomings (Maji n.d.). Research in Pakistan highlights how popular dissatisfaction with physicians has even led the public to seek out wrestlers-turned-bonesetters (Rasheed 1985).

5. The many cultures of the Middle East and North Africa have set the stage for different approaches taken in studies of bonesetters. Some focus on bonesetting techniques and the tensions existing between bonesetters and medical personnel, as in Morocco (Choffat 1979). Others detail the bonesetting abilities of some Turkmen women (Iran) (Maghsudi 2007), suggest that traditional massage may help with chronic back pain (Iran) (Hashemi et al. 2016), or report how in places where Palestinian women's healing roles are changing to emulate men's roles, bonesetters are disappearing (Israel) (Popper-Giveon and Ventura 2009). Cupping therapy, a widespread manual medicine practice, is reviewed from both popular (Yemen) (Abulohoom 2013) and institutional (Turkey) (Arslan et al. 2014) angles. Last, many articles center on the popularity of bonesetters in Turkey (Gölge et al. 2015; Hatipoğlu and Tatar 1995; Köstem and Önal 1990; Sargın et al. 2013) and the medical disquiet it produces.

6. Many works charting the emergence of bonesetting in England and Wales date to the nineteenth century, when divisions between medicine and surgery were sharpening rapidly ("Bone-Setters and Surgeons" 1887; Paget 1867). In this context personnel who thought themselves "qualified" practitioners were intensifying their hostility against anyone they claimed was unfit to treat patients, especially bonesetters ("Doctors and Bone-Setters" 1875). We likewise see legal and medical potentates of the time accosting bonesetters in England ("A Bone-Setter" 1878; Eddowes 1854) and France ("How They Deal" 1887; "Special Correspondence" 1894). Still, the legacy and innovations of Hugh Owen Thomas (1834–1891) ("H. O. Thomas" 1935; Carter 1991; Cope 1995a; Dovey 1971; McMurray 1946)—a prominent bonesetter whose nephew, Robert Jones (1857–1935), became the father of modern orthopedics (Cope 1995b)—occupy much of the literature. Other works document the increasing usage of diagnostic X-rays (Thomas 1906) and UV irradiation treatments (Nicory 1930), trends that dominate the twentieth century. Coverage of local practices and of changing traditions in Wales (Leyson 2004), Denmark (R. Anderson 2004), and Scotland (Bovine 2012) reflects the more localized approaches of later writers, with marked attention paid to the therapeutic benefits of bonesetting in Finland (Hemmilä et al. 2002; Räsänen et al. 2005).

7. Eduardo was very happy to know that I took an interest in his work. Sadly, he died less than a year after we met.

8. I well remember how many bonesetters expressed a willingness to meet with me again during a future visit to Guatemala. My last visit with a Maya bonesetter took place in 2002.

9. B. Paul and McMahon (2001:253–255), however, refer to research showing the prevalence of males or females in bonesetting to be more uneven than this and to vary depending on the community and ethnic group.

10. Hugo Icú Perén, personal communication, 1 November 1995.

11. Gobierno de Guatemala (2010:42). See this source for approximate numbers of inhabitants living in Comalapa's town center and satellite villages.

12. As sparse as the literature is on Maya bonesetters in Guatemala, there exists even less information about non-Maya bonesetters. Writing about Todos Santos Cuchumatán, for instance, Acevedo Ligorria (1986:82–84) spoke of one bonesetter, the only one in town, who was a Ladino. He was said to handle fractures and even inject Lidocaine into joints. This bonesetter kept distant from local Maya curers, but kept close to Health Post personnel (1986:96), perhaps because they were also Ladino. Villatoro (1982), meanwhile, mentioned a bonesetter, possibly Ladino, whom many people would consult in San Benito, Petén. I have only met one Ladino bonesetter in Guatemala, an elderly man who lives in Ciudad Vieja, Sacatepéquez. He applied cupping therapy to me when I injured my back in 1996. Many Kaqchikel Mayas from the area seek his care.

13. World Health Rankings, "Health Profile: Guatemala (health data from 2014 WHO updates)," http://www.worldlifeexpectancy.com/country-health-profile/guatemala (acc. 9 July 2016).

14. World Health Rankings, "Health Profile: Guatemala (health data from 2014 WHO updates)," http://www.worldlifeexpectancy.com/country-health-profile/guatemala (acc. 9 July 2016).

15. World Health Organization, "Country Cooperation Strategy," http://www.who.int/countryfocus/cooperation_strategy/ccsbrief_gtm_en.pdf (acc. 9 July 2016).

16. Instituto Nacional de Estadística, Guatemala (2010:Cuadro [Table] 1.12). ("Porcentaje de hogares por sexo de la jefatura en locales [viviendas] de habitación particulares del área rural de la República de Guatemala en que una o más personas tienen alguna discapacidad, según pueblo de pertenencia y tipo de discapacidad, Año 2002," http://www.oj.gob.gt/estadisticaj/reportes/perfil-estadistico-de-genero-y-pueblos.pdf [acc. 6 May 2018].)

17. World Health Organization, "Health Statistics and Information Systems, Disease and Injury Country Estimates," table 1, "Estimated total female deaths ('000), by cause and WHO Member State, 2004 (a), World Health Organization, Department of Measurement and Health Information," February 2009, http://www.who.int/healthinfo/global_burden_disease/estimates_country/en/ (acc. 9 July 2016); World Health Organization, "Health Statistics and Information Systems, Disease and Injury Country Estimates," table 1, "Estimated total male deaths ('000), by cause and WHO Member State, 2004 (a)"; World Health Organization, Department of Measurement and Health Information, February 2009, http://www.who.int/healthinfo/global_burden_disease/estimates_country/en/ (acc. 9 July 2016).

18. World Health Organization, "Health Statistics and Information Systems, Disease and Injury Country Estimates," table 2, "Estimated deaths per 100,000 population by cause, sex and Member State, 2008 (a)"; World Health Organization, De-

partment of Measurement and Health Information," April 2011, http://www.who
.int/healthinfo/global_burden_disease/estimates_country/en/ (acc. 9 July 2016).

19. World Health Organization, "Health Statistics and Information Systems, Disease and Injury Country Estimates," table 2, "Estimated deaths per 100,000 population by cause, sex and Member State, 2008 (a), World Health Organization, Department of Measurement and Health Information," April 2011, http://www.who.int /healthinfo/global_burden_disease/estimates_country/en/ (acc. 9 July 2016).

20. World Health Organization, "Country Cooperation Strategy," http://www.who .int/countryfocus/cooperation_strategy/ccsbrief_gtm_en.pdf (acc. 9 July 2016).

21. World Health Organization, "Health Statistics and Information Systems, Disease and Injury Country Estimates," table 2, "Estimated deaths per 100,000 population by cause, sex and Member State, 2008 (a), World Health Organization, Department of Measurement and Health Information," April 2011, http://www.who.int /healthinfo/global_burden_disease/estimates_country/en/ (acc. 9 July 2016).

22. Instituto Nacional de Estadística, Guatemala (2010:Cuadro [Table] 5.1) ("Población víctima de violencia intrafamiliar, por sexo, según area geográfica de ocurrencia y pueblo de pertenencia, República de Guatemala, 2008," http://www.oj.gob .gt/estadisticaj/reportes/perfil-estadistico-de-genero-y-pueblos.pdf [acc. 6 May 2018].)

23. World Bank (2013).

24. Having to go elsewhere also depends heavily on people's ability to take or hire transportation, which can greatly depend on weather conditions, especially if they need to take a boat on Lake Atitlán.

25. Gobierno de Guatemala, Ministerio de Salud Pública y Asistencia Social (2012–2016b).

26. Gobierno de Guatemala, Ministerio de Salud Pública y Asistencia Social (2012–2016a).

27. The Asociación de Servicios Comunitarios de Salud (ASECSA) informed me in 2018 that 22,500 midwives are officially certified to work in Guatemala but that these represent only a fraction of the 73,000 midwives working in the country.

28. In recent years, according to personnel at ASECSA, the Ministry of Public Health has imposed more restrictions on what Maya midwives are allowed to do. ASECSA reports that midwives cannot, for example, attend primiparous or even multiparous women (those having twins), at times. Nor can they administer any medicinal plants to their pregnant clients. These restrictions have caused great consternation among midwives.

Chapter 1: Bonesetting over Time

1. Some of these images are available through the image repository of the Wellcome Library (2017).

2. The term *algebrista* appears in Miguel de Cervantes's *Don Quixote de la Mancha*, chap. 15, published in the early seventeenth century. Apart from the *algebrista* mentioned in this passage, Don Quixote's own housekeeper may have also been one, according to Siciliano (1973:387–389).

3. Therapeutic attention to bone among American natives is also borne out in the

North American archaeological record, where we see many skeletons with healed fractures (Goldstein 1957; Hoyme and Bass 1962). In one case orthopedic devices might even be in evidence. A Chaco Period (AD 900–1150) burial in the US Southwest contained a skeleton with a broken radius and ulna; associated with the fracture were six wooden splints (Morris 1924:214–219). This concurs with Ackerknecht's (1947:27) findings that later Native American groups, such as the Creek and Winnebago, treated fractures, and that the Chippewa and Nez Perce even used splints. The Shoshone, furthermore, would make casts for injuries (1947:28). These findings bring to mind Baker (1994), who suggests that Chumash Indians of what is now Southern California used to use *Datura* spp. as anesthesia for bonesetting. This in turn recalls how among Mixe of Mexico, mushrooms and morning glory seeds are ingested as part of the treatment of fractures. They are applied externally as poultices for injuries, toothaches, and burns, as well as for fractures (Lipp 1991:188).

4. Still, in light of lesions found on Lacandon Maya bones of likely Postclassic and colonial date, Cucina et al. (2015:161) comment that "the presence of traumatic injuries and manifestation of *pre*- and *perimortem* cultural intervention indicate hazardous living conditions."

5. He also points to a Postclassic artifact from the coastal El Baúl region showing a human figure with many of its bones and articulations sketched out (Villacorta Cifuentes 1976:129–130), and suggests that its makers had rudimentary knowledge of skeletal anatomy. This recalls fragments of clay figures from Teotihuacan showing a skeletal thorax with what resembles an intestinal volute inside (Dávalos Hurtado 1967:36–38).

6. For translations of the passage on these primordial bonesetters see De León Valdés et al. (1985:136), Recinos et al. (1972:98), and D. Tedlock (1986:93).

Chapter 2: Empirical Forms of Maya Bonesetting

1. Orellana (1987:65) agrees that Maya bonesetters tend not to be explicitly spiritual specialists, even though there exist some mythological underpinnings to their work in the *Pop wuj* (Recinos et al. 1972:98).

2. Whereas in the United States and the West we have medications that are strictly over-the-counter, behind-the-counter, and prescription, these distinctions do not necessarily apply in most of Latin America and certainly not in rural Guatemala. One can buy just about anything over-the-counter where I did my research, including antibiotics. I have generally classed commercial products (including medications) as a single category of products for this reason: they are produced in factories and not in indigenous homes. These products come from a world of organized commercial fabrication, marketing, and distribution that has not had the interests of indigenous people foremost in mind, but indigenous people still buy them and use them on their own terms.

3. Note that some drugs sold as a single brand name (e.g., Mejoral or Dolofin) might be varied in their composition. I found this to be the case from the brand packaging and online drug information from the manufacturers. Different sources can list different base ingredients for a single drug with a given brand name. In different

sources, Mejoral, for instance, might be aspirin or ibuprofen. This ambiguity/inconsistency is pervasive in the Guatemalan drug industry. That said, these drugs, as explained by Guatemalan pharmacists and brand packaging, have the following active ingredients and reported general properties: Indocin (indomethacin [a NSAID—nonsteroidal, anti-inflammatory drug]/analgesic); Anatran (Trichlormethiazide—diuretic—antiedema/antihypertensive); Mejoral (varied: acetaminophen [analgesic], ibuprofen [analgesic and NSAID], or aspirin [analgesic and NSAID]); Dolofin (varied: ibuprofen or acetaminophen); Dolorin (acetaminophen); Dolo-Fenil (NSAID/analgesic/antipyretic); Neo-Melubrina (Dipyrone—analgesic/antipyretic [not approved in the United States since 1977]; Reumetan (indomethacin—NSAID/analgesic).

4. Reumetan is sold in a Comalapa pharmacy owned by a physician. In this pharmacy, the physician's cousin sells this "prescription" drug one capsule at a time, probably with full knowledge of how people take it to relieve symptoms of bodily injury.

5. Icú Perén (1990:48) noted another exception in this regard when he described a bonesetter who had had a revelatory dream.

6. Like Maya bonesetters, Nahuat bonesetters palpate the body with "the sensitive pads of the fingers," probing for the "point" of the fracture or dislocation (Huber and Anderson 1996:29).

7. A Comalapa Kaqchikel man involved in the Pan-Maya movement voices a personal connection to this possibility. He says that it is believed that persons with injuries are destined for a certain curing role and that if they suffer it is because they may be refusing this role. He himself suffers from persistent foot pains, making him think that a healing role is beckoning.

8. In the Nahuat community of Hueyapan, Mexico, bonesetters also use visual criteria when assessing a client (Huber and Anderson 1996:29).

9. One time, when he massaged my back following a suspected intrusion of aire, he applied the pomade Cofal because it warms the skin and "jala el aire pa' fuera" (it pulls the *aire* out).

10. Tomás says casts are "just like a log," and remarks of the injured, "they can't stretch out their feet, the people suffer" from the weight of the plaster, and they are "in tears" by the time they arrive at his house. Despite his tendency to have the patient remove the cast, at least one time he did remove one.

11. To be fair, all bonesetters can be said to have "disgruntled" former clients. I was surprised, though, by how many people disparaged Tonia's work. When bonesetters complained about another bonesetter, more often than not it was about her. When injured clients recalled who had failed to treat them or other people well, they usually referred to her.

12. More enterprising bonesetters might also make marginal profits from the resale of pharmaceuticals, as I discuss in chapter 3 with the case of Lázaro from San Pedro La Laguna.

13. Of note here is the ostensible connection between men and cosmic rhythms, something conventionally ascribed to women (Paul 1984:297). Women are often associated with nature, the moon, natural cycles, and so on. The frequent consignment of women to the domain of the natural (Ortner 1984:73) further operates with the premise that while women are bound up in the domain of nature (and its cycles),

men exist at some remove from nature. The Maya bonesetters' work, however, suggests not only that men's bodies are also subject to natural forces and cycles but that male bonesetters must be especially attentive to these forces and cycles.

14. Tobacco is widely used in the Guatemala highlands in the treatment of fractures (Instituto Indigenista Nacional 1978:276–282).

Chapter 3: Sacred Forms of Maya Bonesetting

1. This account by Lázaro is shown in the original way in which it was written. His way of spelling each word is retained, for example *naci* instead of *nací*, reflecting a personal variation of written Spanish.

2. This Maya use of human bone for healing may hinge on the bone's kindling of regenerative forces in the body's bones. Among non-Maya groups, though, these forces might coexist with destructive energies responsible for disease and directed harm. For example, Mixe associate living bones with pathology and see them as the place where illness resides (Lipp 1991:188). Notably, they also see the bones of ancient sages, from which spring forth mushrooms, as giving people divinatory powers (187). Here, bones set the stage for divination, connecting humans with the knowledge that underwrites shamanism, curing, and possibly sorcery (150–153). Among Rarámuris, this dangerous power in bone can even be externalized and weaponized. Sorcerers of this group reportedly use ground-up ancient leg bones to disable footrace opponents (Merrill 1988:134). Irigoyen-Rascón (2015:122) adds that among Rarámuris, human bones have a connection with death and can cause illnesses in people and animals.

3. Further marking out the instrumental qualities of bone used therapeutically by Yucatec Maya healers is that they also used crocodile teeth and deer antlers when treating toothache (Roys 1976:186, 188, 191).

4. See Acevedo Ligorria (1986:83), Cosminsky (2016:229–230, 233), and Jordan (1989:931) for examples of how researchers have long noted the use of injectable products by healers in the Maya area, especially of oxytocin by some Maya midwives.

5. Interestingly, Lázaro felt no compunction about earlier telling me that a "gringo" had recommended he steep a handful of marijuana in alcohol to use as a liniment.

6. Cipriano recounts that a man from San Juan La Laguna fell from his motorcycle and dislocated his shoulder. A local physician (who was Maya) then gave the man intravenous anesthesia, whereupon the sufferer fell asleep completely. This treatment took place at the sufferer's own house. The physician told Cipriano that he could now manipulate the sedated man. But when Cipriano put his hand on the man's shoulder, he woke with a start, feeling the pain.

7. In these cases, Imelda most likely gives only Neo-Melubrina to the client, and not the combination of Dolorin and Neo-Melubrina.

8. As willing as bonesetters are to incorporate useful biomedical elements, they do not embrace all biomedical materials. In San Pedro La Laguna and San Juan La Laguna, for instance, the bonesetters Lázaro, Cipriano, Imelda, and others readily talk about removing the casts that some clients come with. This is true also of the bonesetter that Clancy McMahon (1994) visited.

9. This merits attention because in other contexts Lázaro recommends using a Coppertone cream because it has a cooling, not a heating, effect. That being said, one person whose foot Lázaro applied this cream to said it felt "hot." These different accounts suggest that the cream has an indeterminate temperature quality.

10. Some injuries are more problematic than others in this respect. Flavio recounted a man who was brought to him from Los Encuentros. This man had fallen into a *siwan* (gorge) in a drunken state and broken some of his ribs. Flavio did not say how he treated the man, but he implied that because the ribs are hard to treat, and because the man was a drunk who was likely to fall again, this case was difficult.

11. *Líquido de res* can be glossed as "beef liquid," and *grasa de toro* can be read as "bull grease." Imelda also calls the bone marrow pomade *"rupam baq"* (the center/core of the bone) in Tz'utujiil Maya. This term for "bone marrow" is also found in the eighteenth-century Coto dictionary of Kaqchikel Maya, a language closely related to Tz'utujiil Maya. Interestingly, the way this marrow product comes from cut bone and is used to treat injured bone seems obliquely homeopathic.

12. When talking about bonesetters in the San Pedro La Laguna area, Rodríguez Rouanet (1969:64) said that they would apply hot *sebo* (fat), sometimes with tobacco, to the fracture or dislocation site.

13. Martín mentioned that Ventura Quiacaín was indeed a *gran curandero*. A friend of the bonesetter Flavio, meanwhile, concurred that although Ventura's descendants have carried on his work with his hueso, one of them is charging too much. Paul and McMahon (2001:253) also describe how one José, a grandson of Rosario's brother, has come to use Rosario's baq, though not without controversy, mostly related to how he overcharges clients. Evidently, compared to his successors, Ventura commanded much more respect.

14. Rodríguez Rouanet (1969:63–64) reported a nearly identical case in which a woman who became a bonesetter after her bonesetter father died would dream of individuals who would then come visit her as patients.

15. Bonesetters occasionally hinted at unexpected lines of transmission, namely, through me. Whether or not they were serious, they considered it possible that I would learn to cure. Victorino said that somebody might injure him- or herself where I happen to be and I will have to cure the person. Then he commented that "Dios yo'on" (God gives [the don]), suggesting that the curing knowledge will eventually express itself, and this will be the outward manifestation of the don. As so often happens in the lakeside towns, the curer shows skill, then the don is confirmed or revealed. Shortly after saying this, Victorino showed me how to wrap a cloth around a hand. Over in San Juan Comalapa, meanwhile, after interacting for several years with Alejandro, he, too, said that I could probably already do some curing.

16. The most active current bonesetters in Comalapa are also over forty, though I cannot generalize for all Guatemalan bonesetters. In San Pedro La Laguna, it is common to find bonesetters younger than thirty or even twenty. In San Pedro La Laguna, bonesetters can accrue prestige even if they are very young. This aspect of the town's practice, though, is probably an exception among bonesetting traditions.

17. The only time a Comalapan bonesetter attributed any supernatural quality to bones was when Alejandro reported the apparition called the *yojlin baq*. Meaning "joined-together bones" (Kaqchikel), the yojlin baq was a being who would appear in the streets as a walking skeleton. It rattled its bones as it walked, frightening un-

wary travelers at night. This skeletal being had an acute supernatural quality because it was "excarnate," unlike other local spooks. This speaks to how Comalapan Maya bonesetters locate sacrality in bone only in rare narrative cases, and only when bone is outside the body. Bones undergoing treatment are never mentioned in such mystical terms in Comalapa.

18. By Orthodox Catholics, I mean those Catholics closely allied with the Catholic Action movement that seeks to move church practices away from syncretic traditionalist expressions and toward an ostensibly "truer," original form.

19. World Health Organization, "Traditional Medicine Strategy 2014–2023," 2013, 52, http://apps.who.int/iris/bitstream/handle/10665/92455/9789241506090_eng .pdf?sequence = 1 (acc. 8 April 2018).

20. World Health Organization, "Legal Status of Traditional Medicine and Complementary / Alternative Medicine: A Worldwide Review" (2001), 58, http://apps .who.int/medicinedocs/pdf/h2943e/h2943e.pdf (acc. 31 March 2019).

Chapter 4: Challenges and Changes in the Injury Landscape

1. As I discussed in chapter 2, many bonesetters from around the region say that they discovered their healing skills when having to fix the fractured bones of farm animals and pets. Physicians take this aspect of bonesetting practice as further proof that the activity lacks sophistication and legitimacy.

2. Clinicians are compelled by the Guatemalan health establishment to form a relationship with community midwives, but they show no inclination to form a like relationship with bonesetters. Midwives, meanwhile, are endeavoring to restructure their relationship with physicians, as their efforts to organize and present a unified front vis-à-vis the medical establishment in 2017 and in other years show (Julajuj 2017a, 2017b; Pocasangre 2017; Sánchez 2017).

3. In Nigeria, as the concluding chapter explains, an initiative has been put forth to train bonesetters as Traditional Orthopaedic Attendants who, it is hoped, will eventually help staff regional trauma centers. This has been proposed because of high rates of posttreatment complications, such as limb gangrene resulting in amputation, linked to the work of local bonesetters (see Onuminya et al. 2000; Onuminya et al. 1999). I should stress that the conditions giving rise to this state of alarm are not present in Guatemala. To the best of my knowledge, Guatemalan Maya bonesetters do not apply tight tourniquets to injured limbs.

4. During this period some orthodox physicians noticed the efficacy of popular bonesetting and emulated some of its features while moving into the bonesetter's professional space, as Cooter (1987) reports for England. Instead of adopting the bonesetter's techniques wholesale, they modified some and excluded others. For instance, Hugh Owen Thomas (Cope 1995a:57), the medically trained son of a bonesetter, felt that while his orthopedic practice benefited from creative mechanical manipulation (long thought a hallmark of bonesetters), it did not benefit from the bonesetters' practice of active manipulation. He argued that rest, not movement, was crucial for successful outcomes. Thomas's views on bonesetters were not typical of the London medical establishment, however; nor did they characterize those

of his orthopedist nephew, Robert Jones, who favored adopting useful techniques from bonesetters (Cooter 1987:167). Another physician, Frank Romer (1915:ix), echoed a dictum offered by Sir James Paget: "Copy what is good in the practice of bonesetters."

5. Notably, even though Dr. Arana says that bonesetters use their hands, he argues that when they treat people, "no hay tracción, no hay manipulación de la fractura" (they don't use traction, they don't manipulate the fracture). He insists that they use their hands only to apply pressure. He also derides how they use the *baq*. Describing a man who fell off a roof and broke his femur, Dr. Arana says he gave him something for the pain, but the man went to a San Pedro La Laguna bonesetter, "y le pasaron el hueso" (and they passed the bone over him), because "creen que con eso, el hueso se va sellar" (they believe that with that, the bone will seal up). He thus considers that rubbing with the baq and pressing with the hands in the absence of other manipulations constitutes the whole of the bonesetters' system of treatment.

6. The purported objectivity and accuracy of radiographs have also been appreciated by researchers of past human groups, who have used X-rays to evince medical and cultural information from bones. Villacorta Cifuentes (1976), for instance, cited X-ray evidence when discussing archaeological Maya bones. He accounted for disease lesions by explaining that early Guatemalans lived an "accident prone life in a constant struggle with the environment" (133). Also examining Middle American archaeological materials, Dávalos Hurtado (1970:68, 73–78) suggested that X-ray analysis could corroborate the specific causes of bone lesions, linking them, for instance, to osteitis or osteoarthritis. Živanović (1982), working in the Balkans, showed that X-rays can help identify the causes of fractures in ancient skeletons, separating trauma-induced fractures from those due to disease or postmortem causes. Other paleopathological works have used X-rays to better evince the etiology of disease and injury (Blom et al. 1933; Brothwell et al. 1969; Saul and Saul 1997). So central have the rays become in identifying trauma that Saul (1972:50) argued "old and very well-healed fractures" in Maya skeletons might go unnoticed if X-rays are not used. X-rays have permitted, and thus mandated, a higher standard of analysis of archaeological bone.

7. Revealing another level of misunderstanding of X-rays, Rómulo talked about how a physician he met in Guatemala City encouraged him to acquire some kind of X-ray glasses. He asked me seriously if such a thing existed.

8. The likening of the hands' abilities to those of an X-ray is also found among Guatemalan Ladinos. An elderly Ladino bonesetter from Ciudad Vieja named Pablo treats many clients, both Mayas and Ladinos. When I asked him (while he applied cupping therapy to me) if clients ever brought him X-rays of their injuries, he said that they did but that X-rays helped him only a little since "my little fingers already know."

9. Farther north, a New Mexico midwife who deals with abdominal disorders is described as being "capable of feeling with her hands what physicians see on X-rays" (Perrone et al. 1989:112).

10. One exception to the pattern of biomedical exclusivity occurs among physicians in China, who have successfully integrated elements of Chinese bonesetting into orthopedics. They found that when dealing with forearm fractures, manual

alignment of the bones and the placement of bone separator pads on the outside of the arm, followed by immobilization, resulted in simple, economical, relatively painless, and effective treatment (Fang et al. 1996; Shang et al. 1987).

Conclusion

1. World Health Organization, "Country Cooperation Strategy," http://www.who .int/countryfocus/cooperation_strategy/ccsbrief_gtm_en.pdf (acc. 9 July 2016).

2. Clinicians in Africa often refer to bonesetters as "untrained quack(s)" (Onuminya 2006:320) or insist that "the peoples' confidence in the TBS is highly misplaced" (Solagberu 2005:108). A. Dada et al. (2009:336) say that "the TBS are dangerous to the society." Ariës et al. (2007:572), however, refer to bonesetters using rather respectful language, suggesting that "bonesetters could further gain expertise in conservative treatment and get the recognition they deserve." See also Owumi et al. (2013:56).

3. Most Kaqchikel midwives in Comalapa today, for instance, are "authorized" by state trainers to practice midwifery, but these women also practice other kinds of physical and spiritual healing that lie outside the allowed parameters. Neither is it likely that Maya healers are limiting themselves to medical strictures in another case: the Guatemalan minister of public health recently said the government would allow certain healers to treat *mal de ojo*, a folk ailment, in certain health posts. It is doubtful, though, that these and other healers have stopped treating people for this ailment outside of these clinics (Pitán 2016).

4. He reports, in fact, that "patients rarely return for follow up [*sic*] when they are doing well," estimating that only 30 percent return (Zirkle 2008:2445).

5. Medical treatment options involving the application of deep friction massage and steroid injections, meanwhile, have shown much promise in the treatment of lateral epicondylitis (Yi et al. 2018).

6. For Mexican Americans in south Texas, an important part of the folk massage experience with sobadores is how these sobadores believe what the sufferers say about what is hurting them. The sobadores do not ask clients to rate their pain on a scale of 1 to 10, or to rate their mobility on a scale of 0 to 100 percent, as is commonly done in clinical settings.

7. The work of bonesetters thus aligns with some of the socially and vocationally driven objectives of occupational therapy. These, according to Yda Smith and Sarah Munro (2008:20), include helping "to facilitate full and successful participation in home and community" on the part of individuals, while placing particular focus on "engagement in occupations that are valued by [the] person."

Appendix

1. World Health Organization, "Traditional Medicine Strategy 2014–2023," 2013, http://apps.who.int/iris/bitstream/handle/10665/92455/9789241506090_eng .pdf?sequence = 1 (acc. 8 April 2018).

2. CMCHK (n.d.).

3. World Health Organization, "Essential Medicines and Health Products Information Portal (Finland), A World Health Organization Resource, Legal Status of Traditional Medicine and Complementary/Alternative Medicine: A Worldwide Review, 2001," http://apps.who.int/medicinedocs/en/d/Jh2943e/7.4.html (acc. 8 April 2018).

4. In this respect, see Organización Panamericana de la Salud (2013:8).

5. World Health Organization, "Country Cooperation Strategy," http://www.who.int/countryfocus/cooperation_strategy/ccsbrief_gtm_en.pdf (acc. 9 July 2016).

6. In this respect, see United Nations (2016:92).

References

Abulohoom, Ali
  2013 "Ancient Practice Continues to Offer Popular Medical Alternative." *Yemen Times*, 20 August. https://www.thefreelibrary.com/Ancient+practice+con tinues+to+offer+popular+medical+alternative.-a0340161393 (acc. 5 April 2019).
Acevedo Ligorria, Joaquín Antonio
  1986 "Una aproximación a la antropología médica en Todos Santos Cuchumatán, Huehuetenango (Estudio de las creencias, prácticas y recursos populares relacionados con la salud)." Thesis, Universidad de San Carlos de Guatemala, Facultad de Ciencias Médicas.
Ackerknecht, Erwin H.
  1947 "Primitive Surgery." *American Anthropologist*, n.s., 49:25–45.
Agarwal, A., and R. Agarwal
  2010 "The Tradition and Practice of Bonesetting." *Education for Health* 23 (1): 1–8. http://www.educationforhealth.net/ (acc. 4 April 2010).
Al-Sulamı, Abd al-Azız
  2004 *Questions and Answers for Physicians: A Medieval Arabic Study Manual by 'Abd al-'Azız al-Sulamı*. Translated, edited, and with an introduction by Gary Leiser and Noury Al-Khaledy. Leiden, the Netherlands: Brill.
Alvar Ezquerra, Alfredo
  2005 "Sobre Cervantes: Vida, muerte, cirugía." *Ars Medica: Revista de Humanidades* 4:4–17.
Anderson, James E.
  1965 "Human Skeletons of Tehuacán." *Science* 148 (3669): 496–497.
Anderson, Robert
  1983 On Doctors and Bonesetters in the 16th and 17th Centuries. *Chiropractic History* 3 (1): 11–15.
  1987 "The Treatment of Musculoskeletal Disorders by a Mexican Bonesetter (Sobador)." *Social Science and Medicine* 24 (1): 43–46.
  2000 "Alternative and Conventional Medicine in Iceland." *Public Health in Iceland*, supplement 2000, no. 1. Reykjavik: Directorate of Health.

2004 "Indigenous Bonesetters in Contemporary Denmark." In *Healing by Hand: Manual Medicine and Bonesetting in Global Perspective*, edited by Kathryn S. Oths and Servando Z. Hinojosa, 5–22. Walnut Creek, CA: AltaMira.

Annis, Sheldon

1987 *God and Production in a Guatemalan Town.* Austin: University of Texas Press.

Ariës, Marcel J. H., Hanneke Joosten, Harry H. J. Wegdam, and Sjaak van der Geest

2007 "Fracture Treatment by Bonesetters in Central Ghana: Patients Explain Their Choices and Experiences". *Tropical Medicine and International Health* 12 (4): 564–574.

Arslan, Müzeyyen, Nesibe Yeşilçam, Duygu Aydin, Ramazan Yüksel, and Şenol Dane

2014 "Wet Cupping Therapy Restores Sympathovagal Imbalances in Cardiac Rhythm." *Journal of Alternative and Complementary Medicine* 20 (4): 318–321.

Atkins, Dorothea V., and David A. Eichler

2013 "The Effects of Self-Massage on Osteoarthritis of the Knee: A Randomized, Controlled Trial." *International Journal of Therapeutic Massage and Bodywork* 6 (1): 4–14.

Attewell, Guy

2016 "Alignments? X-ray Diversions, Haptics, Credibility—With a Bone-Setting Clinic in Hyderabad City." *Medical Anthropology* 35 (1): 5–16.

Baker, John R.

1994 "The Old Woman and Her Gifts: Pharmacological Bases of the Chumash Use of Datura." *Curare* 17 (2): 253–276.

Bali, Yogitha, and John Ebnezar

2012 "Fractures: Ayurvedic and Modern Perspectives." *International Journal of Research in Ayurveda and Pharmacy* 3 (2): 141–149.

Barley, Stephen R.

1988 "The Social Construction of a Machine: Ritual, Superstition, Magical Thinking and Other Pragmatic Responses to Running a CT Scanner." In *Biomedicine Examined*, edited by Margaret Lock and Deborah R. Gordon, 497–539. Dordrecht, the Netherlands: Kluwer Academic.

Barthes, Roland

1982 "The Photographic Message." In *A Barthes Reader*, edited by Susan Sontag, 194–210. New York: Hill and Wang.

Bennett, David

2000 "Medical Practice and Manuscripts in Byzantium." *Social History of Medicine* 13 (2): 279–291.

Berlin, Elois Ann, and Brent Berlin

1996 *Medical Ethnobiology of the Highland Maya of Chiapas, Mexico: The Gastrointestinal Diseases.* Princeton, NJ: Princeton University Press.

Berry, Nicole S.

2006 "Kaqchikel Midwives, Home Births, and Emergency Obstetric Referrals in Guatemala: Contextualizing the Choice to Stay at Home." *Social Science and Medicine* 62:1958–1969.

Bickler, Stephen W., and Boto Sanno-Duanda

2000 "Bone Setter's Gangrene." *Journal of Pediatric Surgery* 35:1431–1433.

Blom, Frans, S. S. Grosjean, and Harold Cummins
    1933 "A Maya Skull from the Uloa Valley, Republic of Honduras." *Studies in Middle America*, Middle American Research Series Publication 5, pamphlet 1, 1–24. New Orleans: Tulane University.
Bolsokhoyeva, Natalia
    2007 "Tibetan Medical Schools of the Aga Area (Chita Region)." *Asian Medicine* 3:334–346.
"Bone-Setter at Fault, A"
    1878 *British Medical Journal* 2 (930): 645.
"Bone-Setters and Surgeons."
    1887 *British Medical Journal* 2 (1386): 198–199.
Bourdieu, Pierre
    1977 *Outline of a Theory of Practice*. Richard Nice, trans. Cambridge: Cambridge University Press.
Bovine, G.
    2012 "The Blantyre Bonesetter: William Rae's Rise to Fame and the Popular Press." *Scottish Medical Journal* 57:103–106.
Breasted, J. H.
    1980 *The Edwin Smith Surgical Papyrus*. 2 vols. Chicago: University of Chicago Press.
Brekke, Mette, Per Hjortdahl, and Tore K. Kvien
    2002 "Severity of Musculoskeletal Pain: Relations to Socioeconomic Inequality." *Social Science and Medicine* 54 (2): 221–228.
Bricker, Victoria, Eleuterio Po'ot Yah, and Ofelia Dzul de Po'ot
    1998 *A Dictionary of the Maya Language as Spoken in Hocabá, Yucatán*. Salt Lake City: The University of Utah Press.
Brorson, Stig
    2009 "Management of Fractures of the Humerus in Ancient Egypt, Greece, and Rome." *Clinical Orthopaedics and Related Research* 467 (7): 1907–1914.
Brothwell, Don, Theya Molleson, Peter Gray, and Ralph Harcourt
    1969 "The Application of X-rays to the Study of Archaeological Materials." In *Science in Archaeology: A Survey of Progress and Research*, edited by Don Brothwell and Eric Higgs, 513–525. New York: Praeger.
Brouard Uriarte, J. L.
    1972 "Médicos, cirujanos, barberos y algebristas castellanos del siglo XV." *Cuadernos de Historia de la Medicina Española* 11:239–253. Salamanca, Spain: Universidad de Salamanca.
Brume, J., and E. O. Ijagha
    1985 "Traditional Bone Setters and Gas Gangrene." *Lancet*, 6 April, 813.
Buikstra, Jane E., and Della C. Cook
    1980 "Palaeopathology: An American Account." *Annual Review of Anthropology* 9:433–470.
Burford, Gemma, Gerard Bodeker, and Jonathan Cohen
    2007 "Traditional Orthopaedic Practices: Beyond Bonesetting." In *Traditional, Complementary, and Alternative Medicine Policy and Public Health Perspectives*, edited by Gerard Bodeker and Gemma Burford, 348–386. London: Imperial College Press.

Burnett, Charles
    2009 *Arabic into Latin in the Middle Ages: The Translators and Their Intellectual and Social Context*. Variorum Collected Studies Series. Farnham, UK: Ashgate.

Car, Glendy, Karin Eder, and Manuela Garcia Pú
    2005 "La herencia de las abuelas y los abuelos en la medicina indígena maya." Chimaltenango, Guatemala: Asociación de Servicios Comunitarios de Salud (ASECSA). https://convergenciawaqibkej.files.wordpress.com/2016/09/herencia-de-las-abuelas-y-los-abuelos.pdf (acc. 27 March 2019).

Carter, A. J.
    1991 "Hugh Owen Thomas: The Cripples' Champion." *British Medical Journal* 303 (6817): 1578–1581.

Cartwright, Lisa
    1992 "Women, X-rays, and the Public Culture of Prophylactic Imaging." *Camera Obscura* 29:19–54.

Chary, Anita, Anne Kraemer Diaz, Brent Henderson, and Peter Rohloff
    2013 "The Changing Role of Indigenous Lay Midwives in Guatemala: New Frameworks for Analysis." *Midwifery* 29:852–858.

Chase, Diane Z.
    1994 "Human Osteology, Pathology, and Demography as Represented in the Burials of Caracol, Belize." In *Studies in the Archaeology of Caracol, Belize*, edited by Diane Z. Chase and Arlen F. Chase, 123–138. Monograph 7. San Francisco: Pre-Columbian Art Research Institute.

Choffat, F.
    1979 "Le traitement des fractures par les guérisseurs traditionnels au Maroc." *Sozial- und Präventivmedizin* 24:172–178.

Clark, William Arthur
    1937 "History of Fracture Treatment up to the Sixteenth Century." *Journal of Bone and Joint Surgery* 19 (1):47–63.

Coe, William R.
    1959 *Piedras Negras Archaeology: Artifacts, Caches, and Burials*. Philadelphia: University Museum, University of Pennsylvania.

Cohen, Mark N., Kathleen O'Connor, Marie Danforth, Keith Jacobi, and Carl Armstrong
    1994 "Health and Death at Tipu." In *In the Wake of Contact: Biological Responses to Conquest*, edited by Clark Spencer Larsen and George R. Milner, 121–133. New York: Wiley-Liss.

Colby, Benjamin N., and Lore M. Colby
    1981 *The Daykeeper: The Life and Discourse of an Ixil Diviner*. Cambridge, MA: Harvard University Press.

Compere, Edward L., Sam W. Banks, and Clinton L. Compere
    1959 *Fracturas: Atlas y tratamiento*. Spanish translation of 4th ed. Mexico City: Editorial Interamericana.

Cooter, Roger
    1987 "Bones of Contention? Orthodox Medicine and the Mystery of the Bone-Setter's Craft." In *Medical Fringe and Medical Orthodoxy, 1750–1850*, edited by Bynum W. F. and Roy Porter, 158–173. London: Croom Helm.

Cope, Ray
    1995a "Hugh Owen Thomas: Bone-Setter and Pioneer Orthopaedist." *Bulletin Hospital for Joint Diseases* 54:54–60.
    1995b "Robert Jones: Father of Modern Orthopaedic Surgery." *Bulletin Hospital for Joint Diseases* 54:115–123.

Cosminsky, Sheila
    1972 "Decision Making and Medical Care in a Guatemalan Indian Community." PhD. diss., Brandeis University.
    1982 "Knowledge and Body Concepts of Guatemalan Midwives." In *Anthropology of Human Birth*, edited by Margarita Artschwagger Kay, 233–252. Philadelphia: F. A. Davis.
    1983 "Medical Pluralism in Mesoamerica." In *Heritage of Conquest: Thirty Years Later*, edited by Carl Kendall, John Hawkins, and Laurel Bossen, 159–173. Albuquerque: University of New Mexico Press.
    2016 *Midwives and Mothers: The Medicalization of Childbirth on a Guatemalan Plantation*. Austin: University of Texas Press.

Cosminsky, Sheila, and Mary Scrimshaw
    1980 "Medical Pluralism on a Guatemalan Plantation." *Social Science and Medicine* 14B (4):267–278.

Coto, Fray Thomás de
    1983 *Thesavrvs verborv[m]: vocabulario de la lengua cakchiquel u[el] guatemalteca, nueuamente hecho y recopilado con summo estudio, trauajo y erudición.* [ca. 1656]. Edited, with an introduction, notes, appendixes, and indexes, by René Acuña. Mexico City: Universidad Nacional Autónoma de México.

Csordas, Thomas J.
    1990 "Embodiment as a Paradigm for Anthropology." *Ethos* 18:5–47.
    1993 "Somatic Modes of Attention." *Cultural Anthropology* 8:135–156.
    1994 "Introduction: The Body as Representation of Being-in-the-World." In *Embodiment and Experience: The Existential Ground of Culture and Self*, edited by Thomas J. Csordas, 1–24. Cambridge, UK: Cambridge University Press.

Cucina, Andrea, Vera Tiesler, and Joel Palka
    2015 "The Identity and Worship of Human Remains in Rockshelter Shrines among the Northern Lacandons of Mensabak." *Estudios de Cultura Maya* 45:141–169.

Dada, A., S. O. Giwa, W. Yinusa, M. Ugbeye, and S. Gbadegesin
    2009 "Complications of Treatment of Musculoskeletal Injuries by Bone Setters." *West African Journal of Medicine* 28 (1): 333–337.

Dávalos Hurtado, Eusebio
    1967 "La osteopatología en los teotihuacanos." *Anales del Instituto Nacional de Antropología e Historia* 18: 35–40.
    1970 "Pre-Hispanic Osteopathology." In *Handbook of Middle American Indians*, vol. 9, *Physical Anthropology*, edited by T. D. Stewart and Robert Wauchope, 68–81. Austin: University of Texas Press.

Davis-Floyd, Robbie, and Elizabeth Davis
    1997 "Intuition as Authoritative Knowledge in Midwifery and Home Birth." In *Childbirth and Authoritative Knowledge: Cross-Cultural Perspectives*, edited by Robbie E. Davis-Floyd and Carolyn F. Sargent, 315–349. Berkeley: University of California Press.

De León Valdés, Carlos Rolando, and Francisco López Perén
  1985   *Popol Vuh: Libro universal de la renovación del tiempo.* Guatemala City: Cenaltex, Ministerio de Educación.
Deuss, Krystyna
  2007   *Shamans, Witches and Maya Priests.* London: Guatemalan Maya Centre.
"Doctors and Bone-Setters."
  1875   *British Medical Journal* 2 (776): 620.
Douglas, Bill Gray
  1969   "Illness and Curing in Santiago Atitlán, a Tzutujil-Maya Community in the Southwestern Highlands of Guatemala." PhD diss., Department of Anthropology, Stanford University.
Dovey, Hugh
  1971   "Bone Setters, Thomas, and Orthopedic Surgery." *Nordisk Medicinhistorisk Arsbok*: 135–156.
Eddowes, W.
  1854   "Two Recent Trials: Seward v. Houseley for Malapraxis; Verdict for Plaintiff; Damages, £250. Crowley v. Thomas, a Bone-Setter, for Unskilful Treatment; Verdict for Defendant." *Association Medical Journal* 2 (60): 182–183.
Eliade, Mircea
  1964   *Shamanism: Archaic Techniques of Ecstasy.* London: Penguin Arcana.
Elliott, C. K.
  1981   "Bonesetters." *Practitioner* 225:253, 255.
Elliott, Iain S., Reinou S. Groen, Thaim B. Kamara, Allison Ertl,
Laura D. Cassidy, Adam L. Kushner, and Richard A. Gosselin
  2015   "The Burden of Musculoskeletal Disease in Sierra Leone." *Clinical Orthopaedics and Related Research* 473:380–389.
Erickson, Pamela
  2008   *Ethnomedicine.* Long Grove, IL: Waveland Press.
Erikson, Susan
  1996   "Pregnancy Pastiche: Ultrasound Imagery as Postmodern Phenomenon." *POMO Magazine* 2 (1): 1–9.
Eshete, M.
  2005   "The Prevention of Traditional Bone Setter's Gangrene." *Journal of Bone and Joint Surgery* 86B (1): 102–103.
Eze, Kenneth C.
  2012   "Complications and Co-morbidities in Radiographs of Patients in Traditional Bone Setters' Homes in Ogwa, Edo State, Nigeria: A Community-Based Study." *European Journal of Radiology* 81:2323–2328.
Fabrega, Horacio, Jr., and Daniel B. Silver
  1973   *Illness and Shamanistic Curing in Zinacantan: An Ethnomedical Analysis.* Stanford, CA: Stanford University Press.
Falla, Ricardo
  1971   "Juan el Gordo: Visión indígena de su explotación." *Estudios Centro-Americanos* 268:98–107.
Fang Hsien-Chih, Ku Yun-Wu, and Shang T'ien-Yü
  1996   "The Integration of Modern and Traditional Chinese Medicine in the Treatment of Fractures: A Simple Method of Treatment for Fractures of the Shafts of Both Forearm Bones." *Clinical Orthopaedics and Related Research*

323:4–11. [reprint of earlier article from *Chinese Medical Journal* 82:293–504 (1963)].

Femia, Paolo
1992 "Los hueseros mazahuas otomíes del Estado de México." *Antropológicas*, no. 4: 60–69.

Field, Tiffany, Miguel Diego, Marua Hernández-Reif, and Jean Shea
2007 "Hand Arthritis Pain Is Reduced by Massage Therapy." *Journal of Bodywork and Movement Therapies* 11 (1): 21–24.

Filer, Joyce
1996 *Disease*. Austin: University of Texas Press.

Flamenco, José
1915 *La beneficencia en Guatemala: Reseña histórica*. Guatemala City: Tipografía Nacional.

Foucault, Michel
1994 *The Birth of the Clinic: An Archaeology of Medical Perception*. Translated by A. M. Sheridan Smith. New York: Vintage Books.

Fry, Edward I.
1956 "Skeletal Remains from Mayapan." *Current Reports*, no. 38: 551–571. Carnegie Institution of Washington, Department of Archaeology.

Gandz, Solomon
1926 "The Origin of the Term 'Algebra.'" *American Mathematical Monthly* 33 (9): 437–440.

Gann, Thomas W. F.
1918 *The Maya Indians of Southern Yucatan and Northern British Honduras*. Bulletin 64. Washington, DC: Bureau of American Ethnology.

Garba E. S., and P. J. Deshi
1998 "Traditional Bone Setting: A Risk Factor in Limb Amputation." *East African Medical Journal* 75:553–555.

García, Hernán, Antonio Sierra, and Gilberto Balám
1999 *Wind in the Blood: Mayan Healing and Chinese Medicine*. Translated by Jeff Conant. Berkeley, CA: North Atlantic Books.

Garrard-Burnett, Virginia
1998 *Protestantism in Guatemala: Living in the New Jerusalem*. Austin: University of Texas Press.

Gobierno de Guatemala, Ministerio de Ambiente y Recursos
Naturales, Sistemas de Información Ambiental
2010 *Información poblacional de Guatemala 2010*. http://www.sia.marn.gob.gt /Documentos/InformacionPoblacional.pdf (acc. 13 February 2014).

Gobierno de Guatemala, Ministerio de Salud Pública y Asistencia Social
2012–2016a "Casos de Morbilidad por Crónicas, años 2012 al 2016." http:// sigsa.mspas.gob.gt/datos-salud/morbilidad.html (acc. 20 April 2018).
2012–2016b "Casos de Mortalidad por Enfermedades Crónicas, años 2012 al 2016." http://sigsa.mspas.gob.gt/datos-salud/estadisticas-vitales.html (acc. 20 April 2018).

Goldman, Noreen, and Dana A. Glei
2003 "Evaluation of Midwifery Care: Results from a Survey in Rural Guatemala." *Social Science and Medicine* 56:685–700.

Goldstein, Marcus S.
    1957 "Skeletal Pathologies of Early Indians in Texas." *American Journal of Physical Anthropology* 15:299–312.
Gölge, Umut Hatay, Burak Kaymaz, Erkam Kömürcü,
Mehmet Eroğlu, Ferdi Göksel, and Gürdal Nusran
    2015 Consultation of Traditional Bone Setters instead of Doctors: Is it a Sociocultural and Educational or Social Insurance Problem? *Tropical Doctor* 45 (2): 91–95.
Gordon, Deborah R.
    1988 "Tenacious Assumptions in Western Medicine." In *Biomedicine Examined*, edited by Margaret Lock and Deborah R. Gordon, 19–56. Dordrecht, the Netherlands: Kluwer Academic.
The Government of the Hong Kong Special Administrative Region of the People's Republic of China, Chinese Medicine Council of Hong Kong (CMCHK)
    n.d. "Chinese Medicine Ordinance" (Cap. 549 of the Laws of Hong Kong). http://www.cmchk.org.hk/cmp/eng/main_faq.htm (acc. 6 April 2018).
Granjel, Luis S. (Sanchez)
    1971 "Cirugía española del Barroco: Traumatología general." *Capítulos de la Medicina Española* 3:121–132. Instituto de Historia de la Medicina Española, Universidad de Salamanca.
Green, Dan
    1958 "Review of *History of Mathematics*, by D. E. Smith." *Mathematics Magazine* 32 (1): 45–46.
Green, Stuart A.
    1999 "Orthopaedic Surgeons." *Clinical Orthopaedics and Related Research* 363: 258–263.
Groark, Kevin P.
    1997 "To Warm the Blood, To Warm the Flesh: The Role of the Steambath in Highland Maya (Tzeltal-Tzotzil) Ethnomedicine." *Journal of Latin American Lore* 20 (1): 3–96.
    2017 "Specters of Social Antagonism: The Cultural Psychodynamics of Dream Aggression among the Tzotzil Maya of San Juan Chamula (Chiapas, Mexico)." *Ethos* 45 (3): 314–341.
Gurunluoglu, Raffi, and Aslin Gurunluoglu
    2003 "Paul of Aegina: Landmark in Surgical Progress." *World Journal of Surgery* 27 (1): 18–25.
Halifax, Joan
    1982 *Shaman: The Wounded Healer*. New York: Crossroad.
Hartouni, Valerie
    1993 "Fetal Exposures: Abortion Politics and the Optics of Allusion." *Camera Obscura* 29:130–149.
Harvey, T. S.
    2008 "Where There Is No Patient: An Anthropological Treatment of a Biomedical Category." *Culture, Medicine, and Psychiatry* 32 (4): 577–606.
    2013 *Wellness beyond Words: Maya Compositions of Speech and Silence in Medical Care*. Albuquerque: University of New Mexico Press.

Hashemi, Mamak, Ali Akbar Jafarian, Shahram Tofighi,
Kamran Mahluji, and Farzin Halabchi
    2016   "Studying the Effectiveness of One Type of Iranian Traditional Massage on Lumbar Radiculopathy." *Iranian Journal of Medical Sciences*, supplement 41 (3): 11.
Hatipoğlu, Sevgi, and Kadriye Tatar
    1995   "The Strengths and Weaknesses of Turkish Bone-Setters." *World Health Forum* 16 (2): 203–205.
Hemmilä, Heikki M.
    2002   "Quality of Life and Cost of Care of Back Pain Patients in Finnish General Practice." *Spine* 27 (6): 647–653.
    2005   "Bone Setting for Prolonged Neck Pain: A Randomized Clinical Trial." *Journal of Manipulative and Physiological Therapeutics* 28 (7): 508–515.
Hemmilä, Heikki M., Sirkka M. Keinanen-Kiukaanniemi,
Sinikka Levoska, and Pekka Puska
    2002   "Long-Term Effectiveness of Bone-Setting, Light Exercise Therapy, and Physiotherapy for Prolonged Back Pain: A Randomized Controlled Trial." *Journal of Manipulative and Physiological Therapeutics* 25 (2): 99–104.
Hernández, Patricia, and Lourdes Márquez
    2006   "Longevity of Maya Rulers at Yaxchilán: The Reigns of Shield Jaguar and Bird Jaguar." In *Janaab' Pakal of Palenque: Reconstructing the Life and Death of a Maya Ruler*, edited by Vera Tiesler and Andrea Cucina, 126–145. Tucson: University of Arizona Press.
Hinojosa, Servando Z.
    2002   "'The Hands Know': Bodily Engagement and Medical Impasse in Highland Maya Bonesetting." *Medical Anthropology Quarterly* 16 (1): 22–40.
    2004a   "Authorizing Tradition: Vectors of Contention in Highland Maya Midwifery." *Social Science and Medicine* 59 (3): 637–651.
    2004b   "Bonesetting and Radiography in the Southern Maya Highlands." *Medical Anthropology* 23 (4): 263–293.
    2004c   "The Hands, the Sacred, and the Context of Change in Maya Bonesetting." In *Healing by Hand: Manual Medicine and Bonesetting in Global Perspective*, edited by Kathryn S. Oths and Servando Z. Hinojosa, 107–129. Walnut Creek, CA: AltaMira.
    2008   "The Mexican American *Sobador*, Convergent Disease Discourse, and Pain Validation in South Texas." *Human Organization* 67 (2): 194–206.
    2015   *In This Body: Kaqchikel Maya and the Grounding of Spirit*. Albuquerque: University of New Mexico Press.
    2018   "The Limits of Conversion: Evangelical Experience and Enduring Maya Principles in Highland Guatemala." *Latin Americanist* 62 (4):568–585.
Hippocrates
    1972   *The Genuine Works of Hippocrates*. Translated from the Greek by Francis Adams, introduction by Emerson Crosby Kelly. [Reprint of 1946 ed.] Huntington, NY: R. E. Krieger.
Holland, William R.
    1962   "Highland Maya Folk Medicine: A Study of Culture Change." PhD diss., Department of Anthropology, University of Arizona.

1963 *"Medicina maya en los altos de Chiapas: Un estudio del cambio socio-cultural."* Mexico City: Instituto Nacional Indigenista.

Hooton, Earnest A.
1973 "Skeletons from the Cenote of Sacrifice at Chichen Itza." In *The Maya and Their Neighbors* [1940], edited by Clarence L. Hay, Ralph Linton, Samuel K. Lothrop, Harry L. Shapiro, and George C. Vaillant, 272–280. New York: Cooper Square.

"H. O. Thomas."
1935 *British Medical Journal* 1 (3866): 259.

"How They Deal with Bone-Setters in France."
1887 *British Medical Journal* 2 (1394): 635.

Hoyme, L. E., and W. M. Bass
1962 "Human Skeletal Remains from the Tollifero (Ha 6) and Clarksville (Mc 14) Sites, John H. Kerr Reservoir Basin, Virginia." *Bureau of American Ethnology Bulletin* 182:329–400.

Huang, Chun-Hsiung
1986 "Treatment of Neglected Femoral Neck Fractures in Young Adults." *Clinical Orthopaedics and Related Research* 206:117–126.

Huber, Brad R., and Robert Anderson
1996 "Bonesetters and Curers in a Mexican Community: Conceptual Models, Status, and Gender." *Medical Anthropology* 17:23–38.

Icú Perén, Hugo
1990 "Práctica de traumatología empírica en el área Cakchiquel de Guatemala." Thesis, Universidad de San Carlos de Guatemala, Facultad de Ciencias Médicas.
2007 "Revival of Maya Medicine and Impact for Its Social and Political Recognition (in Guatemala): A Case Study Commissioned by the Health Systems Knowledge Network." World Health Organization Commission on the Social Determinants of Health. http://www.who.int/social_determinants/resources/csdh_media/mayan_medicine_2007_en.pdf (acc. 29 December 2017).

Instituto Indigenista Nacional
1969 *Santa Eulalia.* Guatemala City.
1978 "Aspectos de la medicina popular en el área rural de Guatemala." *Guatemala Indígena*, vol. 13 (3–4). Guatemala City: Instituto Indigenista Nacional de Guatemala.

Instituto Nacional de Estadística, Guatemala
2010 "Perfil estadístico de género y pueblos: Maya, garífuna, xinka y ladino."

Irigoyen-Rascón, Fructuoso (with Alfonso Paredes)
2015 *Tarahumara Medicine: Ethnobotany and Healing among the Rarámuri of Mexico.* Norman: University of Oklahoma Press.

Jaén Esquivel, Maria Teresa
1968 "El material osteológico de Chiapa de Corzo, Chis." *Anales del Instituto Nacional de Antropología e Historia* 19 (48): 65–77.

Jay, Martin
1986 "In the Empire of the Gaze: Foucault and the Denigration of Vision in Twentieth-Century French Thought." In *Foucault: A Critical Reader*, edited by David Couzens Hoy, 175–203. Oxford: Basil Blackwell.

Jordan, Brigitte
   1989   "Cosmopolitical Obstetrics: Some Insights from the Training of Traditional Midwives." *Social Science and Medicine* 28 (9): 925–944.
   1993   *Birth in Four Cultures*. Revised and expanded by Robbie Davis-Floyd. Prospect Heights, IL: Waveland.
Joy, Robert J. T.
   1954   "The Natural Bonesetters with Special Reference to the Sweet Family of Rhode Island: A Study of an Early Phase of Orthopedics." *Bulletin of the History of Medicine* 28:416–441.
Julajuj, Ángel
   2017a   "Comadronas piden que se frene la discriminación en el sistema de salud." *Prensa Libre*, 8 July. http://www.prensalibre.com/ciudades/solola/comadronas-piden-que-se-frene-la-discriminacion-en-el-sistema-de-salud (acc. 30 June 2018).
   2017b   "Reconocen labor de comadronas en San Marcos La Laguna." *Prensa Libre*, 22 November. http://www.prensalibre.com/ciudades/solola/reconocen-la-labor-de-comadronas-en-san-marcos-la-laguna (acc. 30 June 2018).
Kapur, Malavika
   2016   *Psychological Perspectives on Childcare in Indian Indigenous Health Systems*. New Delhi: Springer India.
Kassirer, Jerome P.
   1992   "Images in Clinical Medicine." *New England Journal of Medicine* 326: 829–830.
Keesing, Roger M.
   1975   *Kin Groups and Social Structure*. New York: Holt, Rinehart and Winston.
Kember, Sarah
   1991   "Medical Diagnostic Imaging: The Geometry of Chaos." *New Formations* 15: 55–66.
Kennedy, G. E.
   1983   "Skeletal Remains from Sarteneja, Belize." In *Archaeological Excavations in Northern Belize, Central America*, edited by Raymond V. Sidrys, 353–372. Monograph 17. Los Angeles: Institute of Archaeology, University of California.
Kevles, Bettyann Holtzmann
   1997   *Naked to the Bone: Medical Imaging in the Twentieth Century*. Reading, MA: Addison-Wesley.
Kleinman, Arthur, and Lilias H. Sung
   1979   "Why Do Indigenous Practitioners Successfully Heal?" *Social Science and Medicine* 13B:7–26.
Köstem, Levent, and Yusuf Ziya Önal
   1990   "Ulkemizdeki sınıkçı sorununa bölgesel yaklaşım (Sivas yöresi anket çalışması)." *Acta Orthopaedica et Traumatologica Turcica* 24:159–162.
Kunow, Marianna Appel
   2003   *Maya Medicine: Traditional Healing in Yucatan*. Albuquerque: University of New Mexico Press.
La Farge, Oliver
   1947   *Santa Eulalia: The Religion of a Cuchumatán Indian Town*. Chicago: University of Chicago Press.

Lambert, Helen
    1995 "Of Bonesetters and Barber-Surgeons: Traditions of Therapeutic Practice and the Spread of Allopathic Medicine in Rajasthan." In *Folk, Faith and Feudalism: Rajasthan Studies*, edited by N. K. Singh and Rajendra Joshi, 92–111. Jaipur, India: Rawat.

Landy, David
    1974 "Role Adaptation: Traditional Curers under the Impact of Western Medicine." *American Ethnologist* 1 (1):103–127.

Le Blanc-Louvry, Isabelle, Bruno Costaglioli, Catherine Boulon,
Anne Marie Leroi, Phillipe Ducrotte, H. C. Sax, B. L. Bass, and M. G. Sarr
    2002 "Does Mechanical Massage of the Abdominal Wall after Colectomy Reduce Postoperative Pain and Shorten the Duration of Ileus? Results of a Randomized Study." *Journal of Gastrointestinal Surgery* 6 (1): 43–49.

Lee, T. Y., and T. H. Lam
    2001 "Mastix is Another Allergen Causing Bone-Setter's Herbs Dermatitis." *Contact Dermatitis* 44 (5): 312–313.

Leyson, Simon
    2004 "A Man of His People: A Concise Ethnology of a Welsh Bonesetter." In *Healing by Hand: Manual Medicine and Bonesetting in Global Perspective*, edited by Kathryn S. Oths and Servando Z. Hinojosa, 237–264. Walnut Creek, CA: AltaMira.

Li-Ming Zhu, Mei Yang, and Feng-Shuang Jia
    2016 "The Traditional Chinese Bonesetting Manipulations." *Proceedings of the 2015 International Conference on Medicine and Biopharmaceuticals* (15–16 August, China), edited by Masahida Takahashi, 169–176.

Lipp, Frank J.
    1991 *The Mixe of Oaxaca: Religion, Ritual, and Healing.* Austin: University of Texas Press.

Lozoya Legorreta, Xavier, Georgina Velázquez Díaz, and Angel Flores Alvarado
    1988 *La medicina tradicional en México: Experiencia del programa IMSS-COPLAMAR 1982–1987.* Mexico City: Instituto Mexicano de Seguro Social.

MacKenzie, C. James
    2016 *Indigenous Bodies, Maya Minds: Religion and Modernity in a Transnational K'iche' Community.* Boulder: University Press of Colorado.

Maghsudi, Manijeh
    2007 "The Native Women Healers of Turkmen-Sahra in Iran." *Iran and the Caucasus* 11:1–9.

Maji, Nirjhar
    N.d. "Understanding and Analysis of the Complications of Traditional Bone-Setter Treatment of Bone and Soft-Tissue Injuries and Their Management in Sub-Divisional Setup." Master's thesis (M.Ch. diss.), University of Seychelles, American Institute of Medicine.

Majno, Guido
    1975 *The Healing Hand: Man and Wound in the Ancient World.* Cambridge, MA: Harvard University Press.

Maoshing Ni
    1995 *The Yellow Emperor's Classic of Medicine: A New Translation of the Neijing Suwen with Commentary.* Boston: Shambhala.

Markatos, Konstantinos, Demetrios Korres, Demetrios Chytas, Marianna
Karamanou, Ioannis Sourlas, Georgios Androustos, and Andreas Mavrogenis
  2018 "Apollonius of Citium (first century BC) and His Work on the Treatment of
        Joint Dislocations." *International Orthopaedics* 42:1191–1196.
Marlin, Thomas
  1932 "On Bone-Setting." *Lancet*, 2 January, 60–62.
Marsh, Howard
  1911 "Bonesetting." *British Medical Journal* 1 (2630): 1231–1239.
Martínez, Francisco Mauricio
  2007 "Sanadores rurales." *Prensa Libre Revista D*, no. 166., 9 September. http://
        www.prensalibre.com/pl/domingo/fondo.shtml (acc. 30 September 2007).
Maupin, Jonathan N.
  2008 "Remaking the Guatemalan Midwife: Health Care Reform and Midwifery
        Training Programs in Highland Guatemala." *Medical Anthropology* 27 (4):
        353–382.
Mays, Simon
  2018 "How Should We Diagnose Disease in Paleopathology? Some Epistemo-
        logical Considerations." *International Journal of Paleopathology* 20:12–19.
McClain, Carol Lee
  1976 "Systems of Medical Beliefs and Practices in a West Mexican Community."
        PhD diss., University of California, Los Angeles.
McMahon, Clarence Edward
  1994 "The Sacred Nature of Maya Bonesetting: Ritual Validation in an Empirical
        Practice." Master's thesis, Texas A&M University.
McMurray, T. P.
  1946 *Thomas and His Splint. British Medical Journal* 1 (4457): 872–875.
Mead, Margaret
  1961 *New Lives for Old: Cultural Transformation, Manus 1928–1953.* New York:
        Mentor Books.
Merleau-Ponty, Maurice
  1962 *Phenomenology of Perception.* Trans. James Edie. Evanston, IL: Northwest-
        ern University Press.
Merrill, William L.
  1988 *Rarámuri Souls: Knowledge and Social Process in Northern Mexico.* Washing-
        ton, DC: Smithsonian Institution Press.
Minor, Jennifer, Miranda Warburton, and H. Vincent Black
  2004 "Achy-Breaky Art: The Historical Development and Contemporary Practice
        of Tuina." In *Healing by Hand: Manual Medicine and Bonesetting in Global
        Perspective*, edited by Kathryn S. Oths and Servando Z. Hinojosa, 81–101.
        Walnut Creek, CA: AltaMira.
Mitchell, Carlton T.
  1989 *Values in Teaching and Professional Ethics.* Macon, GA: Mercer University
        Press.
Mitchell, Lisa M.
  2001 *Baby's First Picture: Ultrasound and the Politics of Fetal Subjects.* Toronto:
        University of Toronto Press
Morris, Earl H.
  1924 *Burials in the Aztec Ruin: The Aztec Ruin Annex.* Anthropological Papers of

the American Museum of Natural History, vol. 26, pts. 3–4. New York: American Museum Press.

Mould, Richard F.
  1993 *A Century of X-rays and Radioactivity in Medicine.* Bristol, UK: Institute of Physics Publishing.

Nandakumar, N., and Goutam Ghosh
  2000 "Herbs Bind Broken Bones." *The Hindu—Folio,* 8 October. www.hinduon net.com/folio/fo0010/00100420.htm (acc. 26 January 2005).

Narangoa, Li, and Li Altanjula
  2006 "From Shamanist Healing to Scientific Medicine: Bonesetters in Inner Mongolia." In *Mongols from Country to City: Floating Boundaries, Pastoralism and City Life in the Mongol Lands,* edited by Ole Bruun and Li Narangoa, 237–253. Copenhagen: Nias.

Nicory, Clement
  1930 "Osteitis Deformans: Its Treatment by Ultra-Violet Rays." *British Medical Journal* 1 (3610): 492.

Nyamongo, Isaac K.
  2004 "Borana Bonesetters: Integrating Modernity and Tradition in a Northern Kenyan Pastoral Community." In *Healing by Hand: Manual Medicine and Bonesetting in Global Perspective,* edited by Kathryn S. Oths and Servando Z. Hinojosa, 221–236. Walnut Creek, CA: AltaMira.

Nyityo, Gabriel
  1990–1991–1992 "Bone Setting among the Tiv." *Humanitas: Man's Past and Present* 7–8:30–40.

Odena, Lina
  1982 *Técnicas de curación tradicional en México.* Colección Xurhíjki 7. Morelia, Michoacán, Mexico: Universidad Michoacana de San Nicolás de Hidalgo.

Ofiaeli, R. O.
  1991 "Complications of Methods of Fracture Treatment Used by Traditional Healers: A Report of Three Cases Necessitating Amputation at Ihiala, Nigeria." *Tropical Doctor* 21:182–183.

Oguachuba, H. N.
  1985 "Mismanagement of Acute Hematogenous Osteomyelitis by Traditional Medicine Men (Native Doctors) in the Eastern and Northern Regions of Nigeria." *Der Unfallchirurg* 88:368–372.
  1986a "Dislocation and Fracture Dislocation of Hip Joints Treated by Traditional Bonesetters in Jos, Plateau State, Nigeria." *Tropical and Geographical Medicine* 38:172–174.
  1986b "Mismanagement of Elbow Joint Fractures and Dislocations by Traditional Bone Setters in Plateau State, Nigeria." *Tropical and Geographical Medicine* 38:167–171.

Onuminya, John E.
  2006 "Performance of a Trained Traditional Bonesetter in Primary Fracture Care." *South African Medical Journal* 96 (4): 320–322.

Onuminya, J. E., B. O. Onabowale, P. O. Obekpa, and C. H. Ihezue
  1999 "Traditional Bone Setter's Gangrene." *International Orthopaedics (SICOT)* 23:111–112.

Onuminya, J. E., P. O. Obekpa, H. C. Ihezue, N. D. Ukegbu, and B. O. Onabowale
  2000 "Major Amputations in Nigeria: A Plea to Educate Traditional Bone Set-
    ters." *Tropical Doctor* 30:133–135.
Orellana, Sandra L.
  1987 *Indian Medicine in Highland Guatemala*. Albuquerque: University of New
    Mexico Press.
Organización Panamericana de la Salud
  2013 *Estrategia de cooperación en el país 2013–2017, Guatemala*. http://iris.paho
    .org/xmlui/bitstream/handle/123456789/5594/ccs_gtm_es.pdf?seque
    nce = 7 (acc. 10 May 2018).
Ortner, Sherry B.
  1984 "Is Female to Male as Nature Is to Culture?" In *Woman, Culture and Society*,
    edited by Michelle Zimbalist Rosaldo and Louise Lamphere, 67–87. Stan-
    ford, CA: Stanford University Press.
Oths, Kathryn S.
  2002 "Setting It Straight in the Andes: Musculoskeletal Distress and the Role of
    the Componedor." In *Medical Pluralism in the Andean Region*, edited by Joan
    Koss-Chioino, Tom Leatherman, and Christine Greenway, 63–91. London:
    Routledge.
  2004 "The *Componedor*'s Place in the Pluralistic Andean Health Care System."
    In *Healing by Hand: Manual Medicine and Bonesetting in Global Perspective*,
    edited by Kathryn S. Oths and Servando Z. Hinojosa, 199–220. Walnut
    Creek, CA: AltaMira.
Oths, Kathryn S., and Servando Z. Hinojosa, eds.
  2004 *Healing by Hand: Manual Medicine and Bonesetting in Global Perspective*. Wal-
    nut Creek, CA: AltaMira.
Owumi, B. E., Patricia A. Taiwo, and A. S. Olorunnisola
  2013 "Utilization of Traditional Bone-setters in the Treatment of Bone Fracture
    in Ibadan North Local Government." *International Journal of Humanities
    and Social Science Invention* 2 (5): 47–57.
Oyebola, D. D. O.
  1980 "Yoruba Traditional Bonesetters: The Practice of Orthopaedics in a Primi-
    tive Setting in Nigeria." *Journal of Trauma* 20:312–322.
Paget, James
  1867 "Clinical Lecture on Cases that Bone-Setters Cure." *British Medical Journal*
    1 (314):1–4.
  1902 *Selected Essays and Addresses by Sir James Paget*. Edited by Stephen Paget.
    New York: Longmans, Green.
Panda, Ashkok Khumar, and Suvendu Rout
  2011 "Puttur kattu (bandage)—A Traditional Bone Setting Practice in South
    India." *Journal of Ayurveda and Integrative Medicine* 2 (4): 174–178.
Pasveer, Bernike
  1989 "Knowledge of Shadows: The Introduction of X-ray Images in Medicine."
    Sociology of Health and Illness 11 (4): 360–381.
Paul, Benjamin
  1976 The Maya Bonesetter as Sacred Specialist. *Ethnology* 15 (1): 77–81.

Paul, Benjamin D., and Clancy E. McMahon
  2001 "Mesoamerican Bonesetters." In *Mesoamerican Healers*, edited by Brad E. Huber and Alan Sandstrom, 243–269. Austin: University of Texas Press.

Paul, Lois
  1984 "The Mastery of Work and the Mystery of Sex in a Guatemalan Village." In *Woman, Culture and Society*, edited by Michelle Zimbalist Rosaldo and Louise Lamphere, 281–299. Stanford, CA: Stanford University Press.

Paul, Lois, and Benjamin D. Paul
  1975 "The Maya Midwife as Sacred Specialist: A Guatemalan Case." *American Ethnologist* 2 (4): 707–726.

Peden, Margie, Richard Scurfield, David Sleet, Dinesh Mohan, Adnan A. Hyder, Eva Jarawan, and Colin Mathers, eds.
  2004 *World Report on Road Traffic Injury Prevention*. Geneva: World Health Organization / World Bank.

Peltier, Leonard F.
  1990 *Fractures: A History and Iconography of Their Treatment*. San Francisco: Norman.

Perrone, Bobette, H. Henrietta Stockel, and Victoria Krueger
  1989 *Medicine Women, Curanderas, and Women Doctors*. Norman: University of Oklahoma Press.

Petchesky, Rosalind Pollack
  1987 "Foetal Images: The Power of Visual Culture in the Politics of Reproduction." In *Reproductive Technologies: Gender, Motherhood, and Medicine*, edited by Michelle Stanworth, 57–80. Minneapolis: University of Minnesota Press.

Peterson, Caroline
  1994 "*Sobadores* as Integral Health Care Providers in Nicaragua." Paper presented at National Symposium on Indigenous Knowledge and Contemporary Social Issues, 3–5 March, Tampa, Florida.

Pitán, Edwin
  2016 "Centros de salud atenderían el mal de ojo." *Prensa Libre*. 23 August. http://www.prensalibre.com/guatemala/comunitario/centros-de-salud -atenderian-el-mal-de-ojo (acc. 18 January 2018).

Pocasangre, Henry
  2017 "Ejecutivo veta la ley que reconoce a comadronas." *Prensa Libre*, 14 March. http://www.prensalibre.com/guatemala/politica/ejecutivo-veta-ley-que -reconoce-a-comadronas (acc. 30 June 2018).

Popper-Giveon, Ariela, and Jonathan J. Ventura
  2009 "Blood and Ink: Treatment Practices of Traditional Palestinian Women Healers in Israel." *Journal of Anthropological Research* 65 (1): 27–49.

Pritchard, Sarah
  2010 *Tui Na: A Manual of Chinese Massage Therapy*. Edinburgh: Churchill Livingstone Elsevier.

Qaseem, Amir, Timothy J. Wilt, Robert M. McLean, and Mary Ann Forciea
  2017 "Noninvasive Treatments for Acute, Subacute, and Chronic Low Back Pain: A Clinical Practice Guideline from the American College of Physicians." *Annals of Internal Medicine* 166 (7): 514–530.

Quinn, Christopher, Clint Chandler, and Albert Moraska
  2002 "Massage Therapy and Frequency of Chronic Tension Headaches." *American Journal of Public Health* 92 (10): 1657–1661.
Rapp, Rayna
  1997 "Real-Time Fetus: The Role of the Sonogram in the Age of Monitored Reproduction." In *Cyborgs and Citadels: Anthropological Interventions in Emerging Sciences and Technologies*, edited by Gary Lee Downey and Joseph Dumit, 31–48. Santa Fe, NM: School of American Research Press.
Räsänen, V., V. Leinonen, and N. Zaproudina
  2005 "Indigenous Healers' Explanations of Low Back Pain and Its Relief." *Pathophysiology* 12:313–316.
Rasheed, Jamal
  1985 "Doctors Ignore Six Generations of Wrestlers Turned Bone Setters." *Far Eastern Economic Review* 129 (18 July): 76–77.
Recinos, Adrian, Delia Goetz, and Sylvanus G. Morley
  1972 *Popol Vuh: The Sacred Book of the Ancient Quiché Maya*. Norman: University of Oklahoma Press.
Redfield, Robert, and Alfonso Villa Rojas
  1962 *Chan Kom: A Maya Village*. Chicago: University of Chicago Press.
Reina, Ruben E.
  1962 "The Ritual of the Skull in Peten, Guatemala." *Expedition* 4 (4): 26–35.
Robin, Cynthia
  1989 *Preclassic Maya Burials at Cuello, Belize*. BAR International Series 480. Oxford, UK: BAR Publishing.
Rodríguez Rouanet, Francisco
  1969 "Prácticas médicas tradicionales de los indígenas de Guatemala." *Guatemala Indígena* 4 (2): 51–86.
Romer, Frank
  1915 *Modern Bonesetting for the Medical Profession*. London: William Heinemann.
Rosenthal, Caroline
  1987 "Santa Maria de Jesus: Medical Choice in a Highland Guatemalan Town." Master's thesis, Department of Anthropology, Harvard University.
Roys, Ralph L.
  1976 *The Ethno-Botany of the Maya*. Tulane University, Department of Middle American Research publication 2. New Orleans: Tulane University, Department of Middle American Research. [Reprint of publication from the Institute of Human Issues, Philadelphia (1931).]
Ruiz de Alarcón, Hernando
  1984 *Treatise on the Heathen Superstitions that Live among the Indians Native to This New Spain, 1629*. Translated and edited by J. Richard Andrews and Ross Hassig. Norman: University of Oklahoma Press.
Sætnan, Ann Rudinow
  1996 "Ultrasonic Discourse: Contested Meanings of Gender and Technology in the Norwegian Ultrasound Screening Debate." *European Journal of Women's Studies* 3:55–75.
Sahagún, Bernardino de
  1974 *Florentine Codex: General History of the Things of New Spain*. Book 10, "The

People." Translated and edited by Arthur J. O. Anderson and Charles E. Dibble. Santa Fe, NM: School of American Research.

Salib, Philip
1962 "Orthopaedic and Traumatic Skeletal Lesions in Ancient Egyptians." *Journal of Bone and Joint Surgery* 44B (4): 944–947.

Salvador Hernández, Pedro Pablo
2011 "La cirugía invisible: El caso de los hueseros Escobar de Cliza (Cochabamba, Bolivia)." *Revista Española de Antropología Americana* 41 (1): 117–141.

Sam Colop, Enrique
2007 "Ucha'xik: Traumatología maya." *Prensa Libre*, 15 September 2007. http://www.prensalibre.com/opinion/UCHAXIKbrTraumatologia-maya_0_149 985060.html (acc. 23 Jan. 2012).

Sánchez, Glenda
2017 "Comadronas denuncian agresiones y exigen respeto." *Prensa Libre*, 5 February. http://www.prensalibre.com/guatemala/justicia/comadronas-denuncian-agresiones-y-exigen-respeto (acc. 30 June 2018).

Sandstrom, Alan R.
1991 *Corn Is Our Blood: Culture and Ethnic Identity in a Contemporary Aztec Indian Village*. Norman: University of Oklahoma Press.

Sargın, Serdar, Ahmet Aslan, Mehmet Nuri Konya, Aziz Atik, and Gökhan Meriç
2013 "Bonesetter Choice of Turkish Society in Musculoskeletal Injuries and the Affecting Factors." *Journal of Clinical and Experimental Investigations* 4 (4): 477–482.

Saul, Frank P.
1972 "The Human Skeletal Remains of Altar de Sacrificios: An Osteobiographic Analysis." Papers of the Peabody Museum of Archaeology and Ethnology, vol. 63, no. 2. Cambridge, MA: Harvard University, Peabody Museum.

Saul, Julie Mather, and Frank P. Saul
1997 "The Preclassic Skeletons from Cuello." In *Bones of the Maya: Studies of Ancient Skeletons*, edited by Stephen L. Whittington and David M. Reed, 28–50. Washington, DC: Smithsonian Institution Press.

Saunders, J. B. de C. M.
1963 *The Transitions from Ancient Egyptian to Greek Medicine*. Logan Clendening Lectures on the History and Philosophy of Medicine, tenth series. Lawrence: University of Kansas Press.

Scheffer, Kathy J., and Richard S. Tobin
1997 *Better X-Ray Interpretation*. Springhouse, PA: Springhouse.

Science News Letter
1938 "Head Hunters Set Broken Bone with Chicle." 33 (24): 378.

Sexton, James D.
1978 "Protestantism and Modernization in Two Guatemalan Towns." *American Ethnologist* 5 (2): 280–302.

Shang, Tian-Yu, Yun-Wu Gu, and Fu-Hui Dong
1987 "Treatment of Forearm Bone Fractures by an Integrated Method of Traditional Chinese and Western Medicine." *Clinical Orthopaedics and Related Research* 215:56–64.

Siciliano, Ernest A.
    1973 "Don Quijote's Housekeeper: Algebrista?" *Journal of American Folklore* 86
         (342): 387–390.
Sierra Hernando, Carlos Hugo
    2014 "Corporeal Transparency and Biomedical Imaging Technologies: A New
         Scientific Imaginary of the Gaze." *Ëa Journal* 6 (1): 1–33.
Sigerist, Henry E.
    1971 *The Great Doctors*. New York: Dover.
Sikkink, Lynn
    2010 *New Cures, Old Medicines: Women and the Commercialization of Traditional
         Medicine in Bolivia*. Belmont, CA: Wadsworth, Cengage Learning.
Simon, Christian M.
    1999 "Images and Image: Technology and the Social Politics of Revealing Dis-
         order in a North American Hospital." *Medical Anthropology Quarterly* 13:
         141–162.
Smith, M. G.
    1955 "On Segmentary Lineage Systems." *Journal of the Royal Anthropological In-
         stitute of Great Britain and Ireland* 86 (2): 39–80.
    1974 *Corporations and Society*. Chicago: Aldine.
Smith, Yda J., and Sarah Munro
    2008 "Anthropology and Occupational Therapy in Community-Based Practice."
         Practicing Anthropology 30 (3): 20–23.
Solagberu, Babatunde A.
    2005 "Long Bone Fractures Treated by Traditional Bonesetters: A Study of
         Patients' Behaviour." *Tropical Doctor* 35:106–108.
"Special Correspondence. Paris. Actions against Bone Setters."
    1894 *British Medical Journal* 1 (1746): 1331.
Spiegel, David A., Richard A. Gosselin, R. Richard Coughlin,
Manjul Joshipura, Bruce D. Browner, and John P. Dormans
    2008 "The Burden of Musculoskeletal Injury in Low and Middle-Income Coun-
         tries: Challenges and Opportunities." *Journal of Bone and Joint Surgery* 90:
         915–923.
Steggerda, Morris, and Barbara Korsch
    1943 "Remedies for Diseases as Prescribed by Maya Indian Herb-Doctors." *Bul-
         letin of the History of Medicine* 13 (1): 54–82.
Steinmetz, J.-P.
    1982 "Traumatologie traditionnelle en Haute-Volta: Étude de techniques d'un
         rebouteux du Yatenga. *Médecine Tropicale* 42 (2): 145–149.
Stewart, T. Dale
    1949 "Notas sobre esqueletos humanos prehistóricos hallados en Guatemala."
         Antropología e Historia de Guatemala 1:23–34.
    1951 "Notes on Skeletal Material." In *Excavations at Nebaj, Guatemala*, edited by
         A. Ledyard Smith and Alfred V. Kidder, 86–87. Publication 594. Washing-
         ton, DC: Carnegie Institution of Washington.
    1953 "Skeletal Remains from Zaculeu, Guatemala." In *The Ruins of Zaculeu Guate-
         mala*, 2 vols., edited by Richard B. Woodbury and Aubrey Trik, 1:295–310.
         Richmond, VA: United Fruit Company.

1956 "Skeletal Remains from Xochicalco, Morelos." In *Estudios antropológicos publicados en homenaje al doctor Manuel Gamio*, 131–156. Mexico City: Dirección General de Publicaciones.

Stoll, David
  1990 *Is Latin America Turning Protestant?: The Politics of Evangelical Growth*. Berkeley: University of California Press.

Storey, Rebecca
  1992 "The Children of Copan: Issues in Paleopathology and Paleodemography." *Ancient Mesoamerica* 3:161–167.

Strowbridge, N. F. and J. M. Ryan
  1987 Inappropriate Traditional Treatment Resulting in Limb Amputation." *Journal of the Royal Army Medical Corps* 33:171–174.

Sweet, Waterman
  1844 *Views of Anatomy and Practice of Natural Bonesetting by a Mechanical Process Different from All Book Knowledge*. Schenectady, NY: I. Riggs.

Taylor, Janelle S.
  1998 "Image of Contradiction: Obstetrical Ultrasound in American Culture." In *Reproducing Reproduction: Kinship, Power, and Technological Innovation*, edited by Sarah Franklin and Helena Ragoné, 15–45. Philadelphia: University of Pennsylvania Press.

Tedlock, Barbara
  1987 "An Interpretive Solution to the Problem of Humoral Medicine in Latin America." *Social Science and Medicine* 24 (12): 1069–1083.
  1992 *Time and the Highland Maya*. Albuquerque: University of New Mexico Press.

Tedlock, Dennis
  1986 *Popol Vuh: The Definitive Edition of the Mayan Book of the Dawn of Life and the Glories of Gods and Kings*. New York: Simon and Schuster.

Thanni, L. O. A.
  2000 "Factors Influencing Patronage of Traditional Bonesetters." *West African Journal of Medicine* 19 (3): 220–224.

Thomas, J. Lynn
  1906 "What Influence Has the Use of X Rays Had upon Treatment of Fractures and Dislocations?" *British Medical Journal* 1 (2366): 1034–1037.

Tijssen, Ingrid
  1979 "Traditional Bone Setting in Kwahu, Ghana." In *In Search of Health: Essays in Medical Anthropology*, edited by Sjaak van der Geest and Klaas W. van der Veen, 111–121. Amsterdam: Vakgroep Culturele Antropologie en Niet-westerese Sociologie Algemeen (CANSA), Antropologisch-Sociologische Centrum, Universiteit van Amsterdam.

United Nations
  2016 *State of the World's Indigenous Peoples*. http://www.un.org/esa/socdev/unpfii/documents/2016/Docs-updates/SOWIP_Health.pdf (acc. 8 April 2018).

Unnikrishnan, P. M., H. P. Lokesh Kumar, and Darshan Shankar
  2010 "Traditional Orthopaedic Practitioners' Place in Contemporary Health: A Case Study from Southern India." In *Health Providers in India: On the Frontlines of Change*, edited by Kabir Sheikh and Asha George, 182–199. London: Routledge.

Urwin, Michelle, Deborah Symmons, Timothy Allison, Therese Brammah, Helen Busby, Morven Roxby, Alicia Simmons, and Gareth Williams
 1998 "Estimating the Burden of Musculoskeletal Disorders in the Community: The Comparative Prevalence of Symptoms at Different Anatomical Sites, and the Relation to Social Deprivation." *Annals of the Rheumatic Diseases* 57 (11): 649–655.

van Soeren, Melanie, and Melissa Aragon
 2017 "The Intersection of Biomedicine and Traditional Medicine in the Peruvian Amazon." *University of British Columbia Medical Journal* 7 (1):60–61.

Villacorta Cifuentes, Jorge Luis
 1976 *Historia de la medicina, cirugía y obstetricia prehispánicas.* Guatemala City.

Villatoro, Elba Marina
 1982 "Vida y obra de los curanderos de El Petén, Guatemala." *La Tradición Popular* 38:1–18.

Walsh, Shannon Drysdale, and Cecilia Menjívar
 2016 "'What Guarantees Do We Have?' Legal Tolls and Persistent Impunity for Feminicide in Guatemala." *Latin American Politics and Society* 58 (4): 31–55.

Wang, Nai-shun
 2008 "Bone Setting Manipulation for the Treatment of Anterior Dislocation of Shoulder Joint." *China Journal of Orthopaedics and Traumatology* 21 (9): 701.

Wanner, Isabel S., Thelma Sierra Sosa, Kurt W. Alt, and Vera Tiesler Blos
 2007 "Lifestyle, Occupation, and Whole Bone Morphology of the pre-Hispanic Maya Coastal Population from Xcambó, Yucatan, Mexico." *International Journal of Osteoarchaeology* 17 (3): 253–268.

Watt, W. Montgomery
 1972 *The Influence of Islam on Medieval Europe.* Edinburgh: Edinburgh University Press.

Wellcome Library (The Wellcome Trust, Ltd.).
 2017 Wellcome Images. https://wellcomeimages.org (acc. 29 January 2017).

Whittington, Stephen L.
 1989 "Characteristics of Demography and Disease in Low Status Maya from Classic Period Copan, Honduras." PhD diss., Pennsylvania State University.

Wisdom, Charles
 1940 *The Chorti Indians of Guatemala.* Chicago: University of Chicago Press.

Wood, James W., George R. Milner, Henry C. Harpending, and Kenneth M. Weiss
 1992 "The Osteological Paradox: Problems of Inferring Prehistoric Health from Skeletal Samples." *Current Anthropology* 33 (4): 343–370.

World Bank
 2013 *Hacia una mejor calidad del gasto: Revisión del gasto público en Guatemala.* Public Expenditure Review, Report No. 78000. Washington, DC: World Bank. http://documents.worldbank.org/curated/en/836891468246600324/pdf/780000ESW0P12300Guatemala0espan00ol.pdf (acc. 31 December 2017).
 2017 *Improving Maternal and Neonatal Health in the Department of Sololá, Guatemala.* 23 March. http://www.worldbank.org/en/results/2017/03/23/improving-maternal-neonatal-health-solola (acc. 30 June 2018).

Wright, Lori E., and Francisco Chew
  1998 "Porotic Hyperostosis and Paleoepidemiology: A Forensic Perspective on Anemia among the Ancient Maya." *American Anthropologist* 100 (4): 924–939.
Yi, R., W. W. Bratchenko, and V. Tan
  2018 "Deep Friction Massage Versus Steroid Injection in the Treatment of Lateral Epicondylitis." *Hand* 13 (1): 56–59.
Yoxen, Edward
  1987 "Seeing with Sound: A Study of the Development of Medical Images." In *The Social Construction of Technological Systems: New Directions in the Sociology and History of Technology*, edited by Wiebe E. Bijker, Thomas P. Hughes, and Trevor J. Pinch, 281–303. Cambridge, MA: MIT Press.
Zank, Sofia, and Natalia Hanazaki
  2017 "The Coexistence of Traditional Medicine and Biomedicine: A Study with Local Health Experts in two Brazilian Regions." *PLoS ONE* 12 (4):e0174731.
Zaproudina, Nina, Osmo O. P. Hanninen, and Olavi Airaksinen
  2007 "Effectiveness of Traditional Bone Setting in Chronic Neck Pain: Randomized Clinical Trial." *Journal of Manipulative and Physiological Therapeutics* 30 (6): 432–437.
Zirkle, Lewis G., Jr.
  2008 "Injuries in Developing Countries: How Can We Help? The Role of the Orthopaedic Surgeon." *Clinical Orthopaedics and Related Research* 466: 2443–2450.
Živanovič, Srboljub
  1982 *Ancient Diseases: The Elements of Palaeopathology*. Translated by Lovett F. Edwards. New York: Pica.

Index

Ackerknecht, Erwin H., 200n3
acupuncture, 31, 191
advertising by bonesetters, 150
Africa, bonesetting in: complications and need for training, 181, 196n3, 204n3; integration with clinical and traditional medicine, 24, 179–183, 192; and radiographs, importance of, 153, 154, 160; repudiation of bonesetters in, 149, 153, 183, 206n2; scholarship on, 6, 154, 197n5
age of bonesetters and status dynamic, 124–125
age of clients: and cold and *aires*, effects of, 82; and healing prognosis, 69–70, 72–73, 74; and injury risk level, 10
aires, effects of and treatments for, 43, 61, 79–84
alcohol, skin application of, 50, 64, 65–66, 80
Alejandro (bonesetter, Comalapa): background and treatment approaches of, 58–62, 65; commercial product recommendations, 43; on dislocation treatments, 45; empathy through personal experience, 48, 49; on lunar cycles, 81, 82, 83; on treating animals, 76; on *yojlin baq* apparition, 203–204n17
algebristas (bone restorers), 30
al-jabr ("algebra" etymon), 30

al-Khowarizmi, 30
al-Qanun (ibn-Sina), 30
Al-Sulami, Abd al-Aziz, 29–30
Altar de Sacrificios site, 35
analgesics, overviews, 43, 96–97, 200n3. *See also individual product by name*
anatomy, understanding of, 28–32, 108, 172–173
Anatran (analgesic), 43, 58
Anderson, James, 35
Anderson, Robert, 5, 125, 147–148, 193
anesthesia, use of, 97, 200n3
animals, bonesetting experience with, 76–77, 147
anti-inflammatory drugs, 43, 72–73, 96–97
Apollonius of Kition, 29
Arana, Dr. (physician, San Pedro La Laguna), 146, 147, 153
archaeological evidence, analysis of, 32–36, 199–200n3, 205n6
Ariès, Marcel J. H., 160
Asia, bonesetting in, 6, 30–32. *See also* China, bonesetting in; India, bonesetting in
Asociación de Servicios Comunitarios de Salud (ASECSA), 9, 20, 139, 141, 191
Attewell, Guy, 54, 160, 177, 193
Ayurvedic framework for healing, 30